Pr

Practical Prescribing

Martin J. Brodie MD FRCP

Consultant Physician and Clinical Pharmacologist,
Western Infirmary and Gartnavel General Hospital,
Glasgow, and Honorary Clinical Lecturer,
University of Glasgow

P. Ian Harrison BSc MPhil MPS MCPP

District Pharmaceutical Officer, Hammersmith and
Queen Charlotte's Special Health Authority, London,
and Honorary Lecturer in Clinical Pharmacology, Royal
Postgraduate Medical School, London

CHURCHILL LIVINGSTONE
EDINBURGH LONDON MELBOURNE AND NEW YORK 1986

CHURCHILL LIVINGSTONE
Medical Division of Longman Group Limited

Distributed in the United States of America by Churchill
Livingstone Inc., 1560 Broadway, New York, N.Y.
10036, and by associated companies, branches and
representatives throughout the world.

First published 1986

ISBN 0 443 03304 8

British Library Cataloguing in Publication Data
Brodie, Martin J.
    Practical prescribing.
    1. Drugs — Prescribing
    I. Title II. Harrison, P. Ian
    615'.1 RM138

Library of Congress Cataloging in Publication Data
Brodie, Martin J.
    Practical prescribing.

    Includes index.
    1. Pharmacology — Dictionaries. 2. Drugs —
Dictionaries. 3. Chemotherapy — Dictionaries.
I. Harrison, P. Ian. II. Title. [DNLM: 1. Drugs —
administration & dosage. 2. Prescriptions, Drug.
QV 748 B864P]
RM36.B76 1986   615'.1   85-20926

Printed in Great Britain by
Butler & Tanner Ltd, Frome and London

Foreword

Each day the general practitioner in the British National Health Service (NHS) writes out 50 scripts (prescriptions). Each year this same general practitioner will spend almost £50 000 of NHS money on prescribing medicines. Prescribing the old 'bottle of medicine' is the most recognisable part of the GP's work. Yet, paradoxically, in the midst of our modern medical advances the quality of our prescribing scarcely matches its huge volume. The GP's training and continuing education are inadequate for the needs of effective use of modern drugs. Moreover, GPs working alone, isolated from the gaze of colleagues, find self-checks (audits) difficult to carry out and apply.

The GP's information on drugs and therapeutics comes from four sources: from publications sponsored by the DHSS, the British National Formulary (BNF), the Drug and Therapeutics Bulletin and the Prescribers Journal; from advertisements and handouts of the drug industry; from reports in recognised medical journals; and from recommendations from local hospital consultants and specialists. All have more cons than pros. They leave general practitioners less than well able to use modern drugs effectively, efficiently and economically.

This is the book that, as a GP, I have been waiting for. It fills many of the existing gaps. The authors have neatly selected out important areas in GP prescribing: choice of drugs for common complaints; policies for treatment; basic information on applied clinical pharmacology; caveats on side effects, interactions and other problems.

It is not the intention of this short book to dogmatise on the use of drugs. The authors seek to stimulate disagreements, discussions and debates amongst colleagues in practice. They offer the book for use in the training of trainees and the education of students. They hope tha it may serve as a work-book for individual practitioners to compare suggestions with their own prescribing patterns.

The Greenfield Report on effective prescribing (DHSS, 1982) noted the need for improving 'training of undergraduates in pharmacology and therapeutics' and also for 'an agreed approach to post-graduate education with a greater emphasis on the teaching of therapeutics and medical management'. This book meets these needs.

Beckenham, 1986

John Fry

Preface

This project came out of a number of sorties into general practice. Monthly lunchtime seminars covering the principles of clinical pharmacology and their practical applications were organised over a period of two years by Dr Bill Styles at the Grove Health Centre, Shepherd's Bush, London. These led me to appreciate the relevance of a grounding in clinical pharmacology to the work of the general practitioner and, perhaps more surprisingly, the acceptability of the message. At around the same time Ian Harrison and I reviewed the prescribing of a single practice in Fulham with the three principals and are most grateful to Drs John Scriven, Keith Fairbrother and Hamish McMichen for their co-operation and forbearance.

These forays culminated in a successful Workshop in Prescribing, organised in collaboration with Dr Bill Styles, which took place in the premises of the Royal College of General Practitioners in London in May 1981. For this event a manual entitled 'General Practice Prescribing' was produced, which must be regarded as the embryo of this project. Following publication of the discussion paper 'Prescribing in general practice: a pharmacological approach' in the British Medical Journal (19 March 1983), more than 400 such manuals were sent out to requesting doctors. Their comments and suggestions did much to stimulate the production of this book, and I am grateful to all those practitioners and trainees for their enthusiastic support. My thanks also go to May Newton who typed the original manual and to Anne Somers for her hard work on this volume.

This book combines an educational approach with much practical material which the prescriber can consult when he has a therapeutic problem. It may be used for training purposes and as part of the normal process of drug audit in the practice. Much of the content is also appropriate for hospital doctors, pharmacists and nurses. It should be regarded as a complement to the British National Formulary and not a rival. Application of the science of clinical pharmacology to the art of prescribing can only result in improvement in patient care.

Glasgow, 1986   *Martin J. Brodie*

Introduction

Over the last quarter of a century, more than 500 new drugs have been released for clinical use. In the wake of their development, increasing knowledge of the mechanism of action and metabolic fate of these and other more established agents has gradually accumulated. In the last decade, improved techniques for dose-response assessment, receptor identification and drug assay have led to a substantial leap forward in the understanding of the ways in which drugs act and are handled in the body. This flood of pharmacological information has the potential to improve prescribing by refining the therapeutic use of drugs with the avoidance of toxicity. To apply this new knowledge the prescriber must appreciate certain basic pharmacological principles. These include dose-response relationships, receptor effects, simple pharmacokinetics and the mechanisms of drug disposition and elimination.

Drugs are potent pharmacological tools. Important therapeutic benefits may be outweighed by potential for toxicity. In combination they may have valuable synergistic properties or produce unwanted adverse interactions. The influence of heredity, environment and disease on drug handling and response should also be taken into consideration. A knowledge of clinical pharmacology must be complemented by an appreciation of the psychology of the prescription and a realistic assessment of therapeutic aim and outcome.

This book may be employed as a practical manual for the prescriber. Its aim is to harness available pharmacological information as a tool to improve prescribing. The first Section is an illustrated glossary of terms providing a concise summary of the pharmacological principles underlying drug action. The next two sections contain suggestions for prescribing. Drugs of choice for common complaints are outlined in Section 2 with appropriate rationales for those choices. The prescriber may see fit to disagree with the emphasis given to some drugs but should consider what he would use in similar circumstances and for what reasons. Empiricism has little place in rational prescribing. Section 3 contains drug treatment policies and strategies for a number of conditions for which chronic drug administration is employed. The broadsheets in Section 4 provide basic pharmacological information for most drugs in clinical use. Sections 5 (side effects) and 6 (interactions) deal with the adverse aspects of prescribing inevitable with the use of all effective therapeutic agents. In Section 7 a number of short monographs under the heading 'Cautions' are brought together.

These include prescribing in pregnancy and lactation, at the extremes of life, and in patients with hepatic or renal disease. A list of non-recommended preparations is included. Some indication is made of the value of therapeutic drug monitoring, and therapeutic ranges for commonly available assays are provided. Finally, there are short pieces on a number of diverse topics from new drugs to shelf life. By necessity there is some overlap between the sections and for this no apology is made.

Throughout this volume, only generic drug names are quoted except for a few proprietary combination products. This will allow easier identification of chemical classes and drug groupings with pharmacological properties and side effects in common, the better to relate them to other therapeutic agents. This is essential to encourage the prescriber to assimilate the appropriate pharmacological information necessary to rationalise drug choice and use. Doctors must be aware of the name and nature of the chemical entities they prescribe. An understanding of the language and principles of clinical pharmacology will take the empiricism out of therapeutics and replace it with a practical basis for prescribing. An index of proprietary products is included to allow prescribers to identify readily the generic equivalent of proprietary drugs.

Frequent review and updating of the composition of this book are envisaged. To this end, user participation and feedback are essential. It is not possible to cover all topics relevant to prescribing in a slim volume and by necessity much is omitted. Additionally the evolution of new drugs and increased knowledge of existing agents will demand change. Your comments on the content and suggestions for improvements are encouraged. A detachable form is incorporated at the end of the book. All recommendations and criticisms will be welcome.

Contents

SECTION 3   DRUG TREATMENT POLICIES   53

SECTION 4   CLINICAL PHARMACOLOGY BROADSHEETS   85

SECTION 5   SIDE EFFECTS OF DRUGS   137

SECTION 7 CAUTIONS

Pharmacological Glossary

Absorption

Although absorption takes place throughout the gastro-intestinal tract, the major site is in the upper small bowel from a surface area calculated to be equivalent to two tennis courts. Lipid soluble drugs are rapidly absorbed by passive diffusion. Absorption of water soluble drugs is slower and may be incomplete. The time to peak plasma concentration is usually around 1 hour unless gastric emptying time is slowed, delaying the drug's arrival to the jejunum. Slowing of gastric emptying can occur physiologically following a heavy meal, pathologically during severe pain such as migraine and pharmacologically due to opiate analgesics, tricyclic antidepressants, antihistamines and neuroleptics. This results in a delayed and attenuated peak drug concentration and effect. Reduction in the rate of absorption is only important for drugs requiring a rapid high peak concentration such as analgesics and antibiotics. Rather surprisingly extensive small bowel pathology, e.g. coeliac disease or Crohn's disease has little effect on total bioavailability of most drugs as compensatory absorption occurs further down the gastrointestinal tract. Absorption of water soluble drugs is more likely to be impaired than that of lipid soluble compounds. Gut oedema in patients with severe congestive cardiac failure may reduce diuretic absorption.

Accumulation

Accumulation occurs when repeated doses lead to a gradually increasing amount of drug in the body. It is a particular problem when the drug has saturable hepatic metabolism, e.g. phenytoin or substantial first pass metabolism, e.g. verapamil. Accumulation occurs to a lesser extent with drugs which have a half-life greater than 24 hours, e.g. nitrazepam although with these the attainment of steady-state around five half-lives after initiation of therapy limits the rise in drug concentration (Fig. 1.1). As drug elimination is slower in the elderly, accumulation occurs more often.

Antagonism

Drugs acting on the same biological system may antagonise one another's pharmacological effects. This can be used therapeutically as in the treatment of opiate poisoning with naloxone. Obvious antagonisms are easily avoided such as a thiazide diuretic in a diabetic patient receiving an oral hypoglycaemic agent. Some are less easily predicted such as the antagonism of the blood pressure lowering effects of beta blockers by non-steroidal anti-inflammatory agents which suggests a local renal prostaglandin mediated mechanism of action for these antihypertensive drugs.

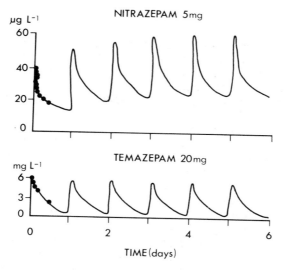

Fig. 1.1 Comparison of plasma levels of nitrazepam (half-life 36 hours) and temazepam (half-life 8 hours) following repeated evening dozes. Nitrazepam accumulates during the day

Biliary excretion

Lipid-soluble drugs may be excreted in the bile. They are occasionally eliminated unchanged but most often as the conjugated metabolite. Biliary excretion also provides a 'back-up' method of elimination when renal function is impaired. Reabsorption in the ileum may provide an enterohepatic cycle which may prolong a drug's action. Metabolites may be deconjugated by intestinal bacteria and the parent drug reabsorbed. This occurs with some benzodiazepines and may increase the duration of their pharmacological effect. A similar mechanism operates with the components of the oral contraceptive pill and disruption of this enterohepatic circulation by broad-spectrum antibiotics which eliminate the deconjugating bacteria may reduce circulating hormone concentrations and result in contraceptive failure.

Bioavailability

This is the term used to describe the percentage of an oral dose reaching the systemic circulation. It depends on the extent of absorption of the drug and the amount metabolised on the 'first pass' through the gut wall and liver. As drug injected intravenously is 100% bioavailable, it is calculated as the ratio of the areas under the oral and intravenous concentration-time curves following a single drug dose given by both routes (Fig. 1.2). Similar bioavailability calculations can be made for topical or rectal formulations.

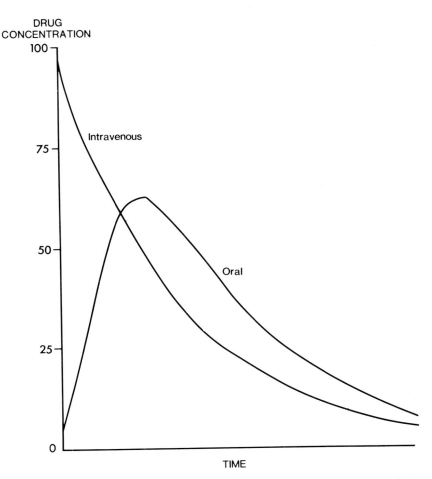

DRUG
CONCENTRATION

Fig. 1.2 Superimposed concentration-time curves for the same dose of a drug given intravenously and orally. The bioavailability is calculated as the ratio of the area under the oral curve as a percentage of the intravenous. In this case bioavailability approximates to 100%

Bioavailability of a drug given chronically may differ from that calculated following a single dose. The total amount of available drug is less important than the variation in its bioavailability. It is this variation which makes drugs with a high first pass metabolism particularly difficult to prescribe effectively.

Blood brain barrier

The blood brain barrier consists of tight junctions between the endothelial cells of the cerebral capillaries, choroid plexuses and arachnoid villi. Drugs must cross this to gain access to the cerebrospinal fluid and neurones. Lipid soluble drugs reach the brain readily and if given intravenously, e.g. diazepam, can produce an effect within a minute. Water soluble substances such as penicillin and some cytotoxic drugs have little access to the brain and may require to be administered intrathecally. Thus the lipid soluble beta blocker propranolol may produce vivid dreams whereas the water soluble atenolol is much less likely to do so. The selectivity of the blood brain barrier is utilised therapeutically in the treatment of Parkinsonism in preparations containing levodopa and a dopa decarboxylase inhibitor (Sinemet, Madopar). The inhibitor prevents the peripheral breakdown of levodopa but does not cross the blood brain barrier itself and therefore does not influence the therapeutic action of levodopa in the basal ganglia.

Clearance

Clearance is the most accurate measure of drug elimination. It is obtained by dividing the dose administered by the area under the concentration-time curve and is usually expressed as the volume of plasma cleared of drug per unit time, e.g. ml/min as for creatinine clearance. Drug clearance is often a composite of renal and hepatic clearances and is the most precise parameter for kinetic comparisons as it is not dependent on the volume of distribution. It is of little value in the clinical situation and is largely employed in research.

Distribution

The distribution of a drug is its reversible transfer throughout the plasma, extracellular fluid and tissues after it has been injected or absorbed. The volume of distribution is a convenient mathematical term which assumes that the drug is present throughout the body in the same concentration as in the plasma. It is calculated in litres by dividing an intravenous dose by the estimated drug concentration at the time of injection (Co). Co is calculated from a log-linear concentration time curve as in Fig. 1.3. It gives some measure of the amount of a drug load remaining in the plasma and that bound in the tissue. Thus if all the drug is confined to the vascular compartment the volume of distribution would be around 5 litres. Many drugs, such as amitriptyline, have volumes of distribution over 250 litres, suggesting that most of the drug leaves the plasma and is bound in the tissues.

Dose response

Each pharmacodynamic response to a drug can be related to its concentration at the site of action and, therefore, the dose

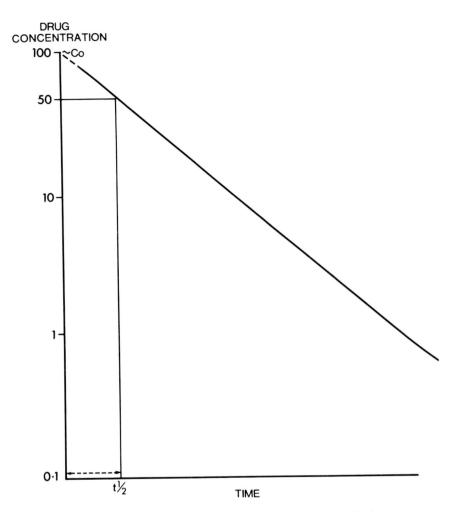

Fig. 1.3 Concentration-time curve for a drug given intravenously with the concentration plotted on a logarithmic scale. For most drugs this results in a straight line. The estimated plasma concentration at the time of injection (Co) can be obtained by extrapolating the line backwards to the vertical axis— in this case 100 units. Volume of distribution can then be calculated as the dose/Co. The half-life ($t\frac{1}{2}$) of the drug can be read off as the time taken for the concentration to fall by half, e.g. from 100 to 50 units

administered. There is a minimum dose at which an effect is detectable and another where maximal change is produced above which no further increase is possible (Fig. 1.4). By plotting the dose on a logarithmic scale, the typical S-shaped curve is obtained (Fig. 1.5). The dose-response curve for the same drug may differ substantially between individual patients. Generally, drugs with a flat dose-response curve, e.g. atenolol, are easier to use clinically than those with a steep dose-response curve, e.g. methlydopa (Fig. 1.6),

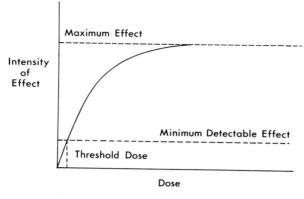

Fig. 1.4 Simple dose-response curve plotting dose against intensity of effect. For each drug there is a threshold dose at which an effect can be detected and a maximum dose above which no increase in effect can be produced

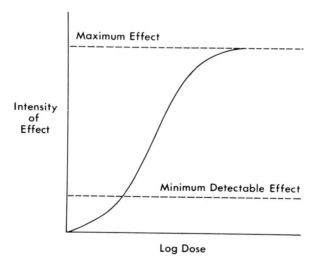

Fig. 1.5 Classical S-shaped dose-response curve obtained by plotting the dose on a logarithmic scale against intensity of effect. The potency of the drug can be obtained by considering its position on the horizontal axis and the efficacy as the percentage of maximum effect obtained

as fewer dosage increments are needed and side-effects are less likely to be a problem. The dose-response curves for side-effects must also be considered. Thus 5 mg of bendrofluazide is the maximal hypotensive dose of the drug. Higher doses produce the same fall in blood pressure but greater long-term toxicity, e.g. hypokalaemia, hyperuricaemia, hyperglycaemia, hyperlipidaemia. However, the dose-response to the diuretic effect of bendrofluazide is steeper and 10 mg will produce an increased diuresis.

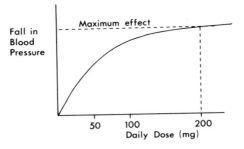

FLAT e.g. ATENOLOL

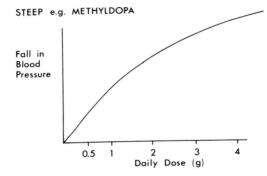

STEEP e.g. METHYLDOPA

Fig. 1.6 Comparison of simple dose-response curves for atenolol and methyldopa. An atenolol dose of around 200 mg will produce the maximum hypotensive effect whereas increasing doses of methyldopa will extend its hypotensive action and potential for toxicity

Drug allergy

There are a number of ways in which an allergic reaction to a drug can produce tissue damage or disease. The best known and probably most feared is the immediate anaphylactic reaction to venoms, vaccines, blood products and parenterally administered drugs. The allergen reacts with tissue cells releasing pharmacological mediators such as histamine, kinins and prostaglandins resulting in increased vascular permeability and contraction of smooth muscle. This type I reaction is also implicated in the pathogenesis of angioneurotic oedema, hay fever, urticaria and asthma. Treatment aims to block the pharmacological effects of the released substances with adrenaline, corticosteroids and antihistamines. In type II reactions antibody to a drug reacts with an antigenic component on the cell. Complement is usually consumed and a cytotoxic reaction produced, e.g. haemolytic anaemia (sulphonamides) and thrombocytopenic purpura (quinine). Treatment with corticosteroids usually ameliorates the condition. The Arthus (type III) reaction is a consequence of damage due to circulating antigen-antibody complexes. This can produce an illness resembling serum sickness with fever, arthralgia, rash and lymphadenopathy. The onset occurs 7–12 days after initiating the offending agent and is most commonly seen with penicillins, aspirin and sulphonamides. Rarely, an SLE-like syndrome can occur (hydralazine, phenytoin, methyldopa, procainamide). Once again withdrawal of the toxic drug and treatment with corticosteroids will produce remission. Delayed (type IV) hypersensitivity occurs when lymphocytes become sensitised to a drug. This mechanism is responsible for most instances of contact dermatitis. All allergic drug reactions are idiosyncratic (type B) and more than one immunological mechanism may be involved.

Elimination

Drug elimination represents its irreversible loss from the body, largely by metabolism in the liver, excretion by the kidneys or a combination of both. Drug metabolites are excreted in the bile and urine.

Enzyme induction

A few drugs bind to cytosolic cellular receptors in the liver and other organs to trigger the increased production of metabolic enzymes. As protein synthesis is required the maximum effect is not apparent for 2–3 weeks. The result is increased metabolism of a number of drugs and endogenous hormones eliminated by the liver with reduction in their circulating levels and attenuation of their pharmacological effects. The most potent enzyme inducers are rifampicin, phenobarbitone, phenytoin and carbamazepine. Other drugs also have enzyme-inducing properties (Table 1.1). Important interactions can occur particularly with drugs with a narrow therapeutic ratio such as corticosteroids, oral contraceptives, warfarin, opiates and cardiac antiarrhythmics and demand an increased dose of the induced drug. When the inducing agent is withdrawn, the process is reversed and toxic levels of induced drug may be produced unless Its dose is reduced. Carbamazepine can induce its own metabolism with a fall off in plasma concentration on an unchanged dose and consequent reduction in anticonvulsant efficacy.

Table 1.1 Enzyme inducers in clinical use

Barbiturates	Marijuana smoke
Carbamazepine	Meprobamate
Cigarette smoke	Phenobarbitone
Dichloralphenazone	Phenytoin
Ethanol (Chronic)	Primidone (Phenobarbitone)
Glutethimide	Rifampicin
Griseofulvin	Sulphinpyrazone

Enzyme inhibition

Lipid-soluble drugs can have their hepatic metabolism inhibited by other drugs. This produces an increase in plasma level of the inhibited drug, maximal five half-lives later, when a new steady-state is produced. Maximal potentiation of the pharmacological effect of a drug with a short half-life like tolbutamide may occur in 24–48 hours. Inhibition of the metabolism of a drug with a long half-life such as warfarin may not be complete for a week or more. When an inhibition interaction is recognised, the inhibitor may be discontinued or the dose of the target drug reduced. Many commonly used drugs have inhibitory properties (Table 1.2) but the degree of interaction and extent of the clinical effect varies between individual patients and is, therefore, unpredictable. When an inhibiting drug is withdrawn the plasma concentration of the target drug will fall with some reduction in its therapeutic effect. Enzyme inhibitors should be avoided if possible in patients receiving chronic therapy with a number of lipid-soluble drugs and, in particular, those with a narrow therapeutic ratio such as warfarin, phenytoin and theophylline.

Table 1.2   Enzyme inhibitors in clinical use

Allopurinol	Metronidazole
Amiodarone	Miconazole
Azapropazone	Nortriptyline
Chloramphenicol	Oral contraceptives
Chlorpromazine	Oxyphenbutazone
Cimetidine	Perphenazine
Dextropropoxyphene	Phenylbutazone
Disulfiram	Primaquine
Ethanol (Acute)	Propranolol
Erythromycin	Sodium valproate
Imipramine	Sulphinpyrazone
Isoniazid	Sulphonamides
Ketoconazole	Thioridazine
Metoprolol	

First pass metabolism

A number of drugs when given orally undergo substantial metabolism on the first pass through the gut wall, liver or both (Table 1.3). As a result less than 50% of a single oral dose reaches the systemic circulation and its site of action. Because this metabolism is saturable, a 40-fold variation in peak plasma concentration may

Table 1.3 Drugs undergoing substantial first pass metabolism

Cardiac	Analgesic
Glyceryl trinitrate	Aspirin
Hydralazine	Codeine
Indoramin	Dextropropoxyphene
Isoprenaline	Meptazinol
Isosorbide dinitrate	Morphine
Labetalol	Pentazocine
Lignocaine	Pethidine
Metoprolol	
Prazosin	
Propranolol	**Psychiatric**
Verapamil	Amitriptyline
	Chlormethiazole
	Chlorpromazine
Respiratory	Doxepin
Salbutamol	Imipramine
Terbutaline	Methylphenidate
	Nortriptyline
Neurological	
Dihydroergotamine	**Cytotoxic**
Levodopa	Fluorouracil
Neostigmine	Mercaptopurine
Others	
Domperidone	
Oral contraceptives	
Praziquantel	

occur following the same oral dose given to a number of patients. On chronic dosing, steady-state levels are higher than expected and may vary 5-fold. In patients with hepatic cirrhosis by-passing of hepatic metabolism by porto-systemic shunting will markedly increase the bioavailability of these drugs. In such patients peak plasma levels may be as much as five times that occurring in patients with normal liver function receiving the same dose. Care must then be taken in prescribing high first pass drugs for cirrhotics and also for the elderly in whom first pass metabolism is also reduced.

Half-life

The half-life represents the time taken for the drug concentration in the plasma to fall by half. When a drug is given intravenously and blood removed frequently over the next few hours for drug assay a concentration-time curve can be constructed as in Fig. 1.7. For most drugs the amount eliminated from the plasma is directly proportional to the amount present, i.e. first order kinetics, and so if the concentration is plotted on a logarithmic scale, the original curve becomes a straight line from which the elimination half-life can be easily read off as in Fig. 1.3. The concentration time curve following an oral dose is more complicated as the drug must be absorbed and distributed throughout the tissues prior to metabolism or excretion (Fig. 1.8). Once again, however, when the concentration is plotted on a logarithmic scale, the declining part of the curve will usually be a straight line and the 'elimination' half-life readily obtained.

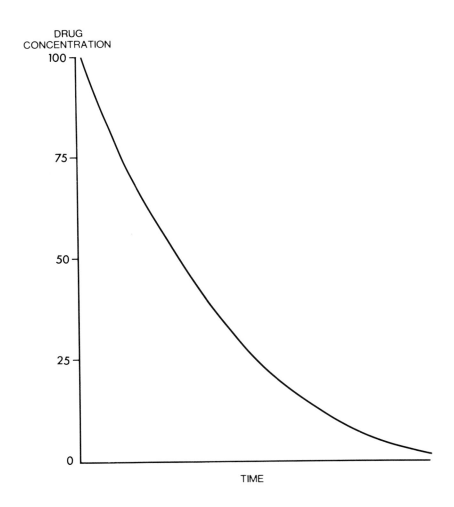

Fig. 1.7 Simple concentration-time curve for a drug given intravenously

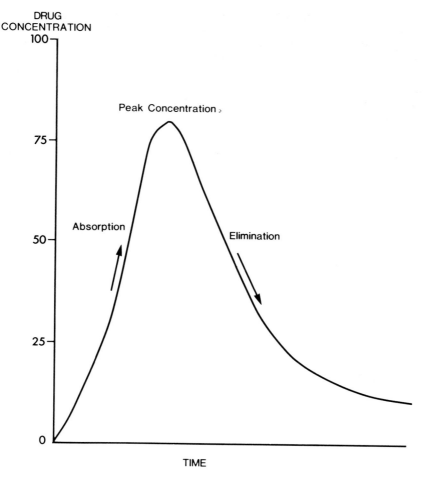

Fig. 1.8 Concentration-time curve following an oral dose of a drug. A delay occurs in the peak concentration depending on the time taken for absorption and distribution. This peak may be further delayed and reduced with concomitant administration of a drug which reduces gastric emptying, e.g. tricyclic antidepressant. The steepness of the downslope is a function of the rate of elimination of the drug, i.e. the elimination half-life

Hypersensitivity

Hypersensitivity occurs when an unexpectedly substantial response is apparent following a relatively modest dose of a drug. A hypersensitivity phenomenon may also be produced to endogenous substances when a drug is withdrawn due to changes in receptor numbers. Long-term treatment with an antagonist, e.g. a beta blocker, results in an increased number of receptors to the endogenous agonist, in this case noradrenaline and adrenaline. This 'up-regulation' of receptor numbers can produce a hypersensitivity effect when the antagonist is withdrawn. Examples of this phenomenon include tardive dyskinesia with phenothiazines (dopaminergic antagonists) probably due to increased numbers of dopamine receptors and rebound angina and myocardial infarction following propranolol (beta adrenoceptor antagonist) withdrawal. Sudden discontinuation of some agonist drugs such as opiates and benzodiazepines may also cause a withdrawal syndrome and this may be a function of excessive release of other neurotransmitters such as noradrenaline. Drugs binding to receptors should always be reduced slowly and never suddenly discontinued.

Idiosyncratic adverse effects

Rarely a drug will produce a severe and often fatal idiosyncratic reaction such as aplastic anaemia, hepatotoxicity or acute renal failure. These effects are not dose-dependent and are completely unpredictable. This type of adverse reaction is also known as a type B reaction and occurs in less than 1:10 000 patients receiving the drug. By their very rarity they may be unavoidable. If the drug concerned is one of many available for the same indication, such an adverse effect, however rare, may be unacceptable and the drug may be withdrawn, e.g. aplastic anaemia with phenylbutazone and oxyphenbutazone.

Inhalers

Drugs given by inhalation may produce a local effect in the lungs, e.g. salbutamol and beclomethasone in asthma, with doses low enough to avoid systemic effects. This route may also be of value in producing a rapid pharmacological response with drugs undergoing substantial first pass metabolism, e.g. glyceryl trinitrate in angina, ergotamine tartrate in migraine.

Intramuscular injection

Intramuscular drug administration rarely conveys any clinical advantage. The muscle may act as a trap out of which drug leaks over many hours and bioavailability is often unpredictable. Peak concentrations may be delayed. Some drugs such as phenytoin may even crystallise out in muscle. These properties may be employed usefully as depot preparations, e.g. flupenthixol in schizophrenia. If an immediate effect is required, the intravenous route is usually preferred. If not, most drugs given orally will reach their peak concentration in 30–120 minutes. Exceptions occur with a few drugs insufficiently absorbed orally such as the aminoglycoside antibiotics and gold preparations which require parenteral administration.

Intravenous injection

Following an intravenous bolus, drug is rapidly distributed throughout the body and its pharmacological effect may be apparent in minutes. To allow distribution to proceed rapidly but with avoidance of very high plasma concentrations, all intravenous drugs should be given slowly over several minutes or diluted in saline or dextrose and infused over 15–20 minutes. In the hospital setting, a longer intravenous infusion may be preferred with monitoring of plasma levels, e.g. theophylline in severe asthma or phenytoin in status epilepticus.

Lipid soluble drugs

The majority of drugs in clinical use are lipid soluble requiring metabolism, usually in the liver, to more water soluble substances which are then excreted in bile and/or urine. Lipid soluble drugs are rapidly absorbed and quickly reach their site of action. They readily cross the blood-brain barrier, placenta and breast epithelium. Dosage reduction may be required in patients with hepatic cirrhosis, particularly if the drug has a narrow therapeutic ratio.

Loading dose

As it takes around five half-lives for a drug to attain steady-state, a week or more may elapse before this is achieved for drugs with long half-lives such as digoxin and warfarin. In some instances a loading dose may be administered to offset this delay in obtaining satisfactory plasma concentrations. The amount of the loading dose is a function of the volume of distribution of the drug, i.e. the amount required to saturate tissue binding sites. As a general rule, the loading dose is usually 2–3 times the maintenance dose, e.g. 0.5–0.75 mg for digoxin.

Metabolism

Most drugs are lipid soluble and require to be transformed to more water soluble products prior to excretion in the bile or urine. The liver is the major metabolic factory of the body. The metabolism of many drugs requires two separate phases — oxidation and conjugation (Fig. 1.9). The phase 1 enzymes responsible for oxidation and similar reactions are known as monooxygenases and can be collectively measured in liver tissue as cytochrome P_{450}. The metabolites produced are usually inert but may have biological activity, although this is usually less than for the parent compound. Rarely a toxic (e.g. following paracetamol overdose) or even carcinogenic (e.g. from cigarette smoke) substance can be formed. Some pro-drugs (e.g. cyclophosphamide, sulindac) require to be metabolised to produce

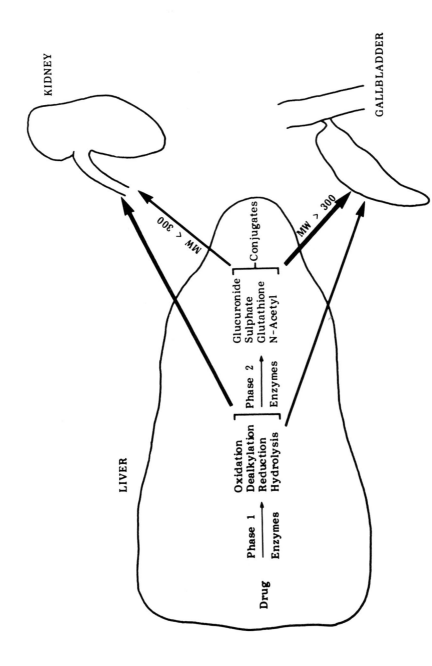

Fig. 1.9 Hepatic metabolic routes for lipid-soluble drugs. Metabolism may be by phase 1 (oxidation and similar reactions) and/or phase 2 (conjugating) enzymes. Metabolites are eliminated in the bile and/or urine

the active agent. Products of oxidation reactions may be excreted directly or further metabolised by phase 2 enzymes. This involves the addition of an endogenous substance such as sulphate or glucuronic acid to produce a conjugate. Some drugs are metabolised only by conjugation. Almost all conjugates are inert. The larger molecules are excreted in the bile whereas the smaller ones (molecular weight less than 300) also pass out in the urine. Premature infants have impaired drug metabolism whereas infants and young children may eliminate lipid soluble drugs more rapidly than adults. Thereafter, the activity of these enzymes gradually tails off into old age. Dosage adjustment of lipid soluble drugs in liver disease is crude as impairment of hepatic metabolic function correlates poorly with biochemical liver function tests. Patients with proven cirrhosis should be prescribed initially half the standard dose of a drug primarily eliminated by oxidation processes. Conjugated drugs can be given in standard doses until clinical signs of hepatic decompensation, such as ascites and pre-coma, supervene.

Peak and trough concentrations

The steady-state concentration of a drug represents the average value throughout the day. Clearly the concentration will vary as new drug is absorbed and circulating drug metabolised and excreted. This results in a number of peaks and troughs depending on the number of daily doses. The height of peaks and depth of troughs will then depend on the half-life of the drug concerned and the number of doses administered (Fig. 1.10). Thus, although for some drugs with a half-life greater than 24 hours, such as phenobarbitone, a single daily dose would provide an acceptable steady-state concentration, it would also produce a high peak concentration several hours after the dose which may result in unacceptable sedation. Splitting the dose into a number of smaller increments may be preferred, although this may result in poorer compliance. Conversely, when an aminoglycoside antibiotic is prescribed, a high peak concentration is desirable to eradicate the organism but a low trough is necessary to avoid damage to the inner ear and kidney. Thus, with gentamicin a large dose is given as infrequently as possible. For most drugs high peaks and low troughs are best avoided and a true steady-state with no hour-to-hour variation would be ideal. This can only be achieved by an intravenous infusion. However, this unattainable aim is responsible for the plethora of slow-release preparations currently available. The other theoretical advantage of these is improved compliance. A short acting drug with a narrow therapeutic ratio and a good concentration-effect relationship such as theophylline is ideal for this approach. Clearly it is unlikely to be appropriate for a drug with a half-life greater than 24 hours such as amitriptyline or diazepam.

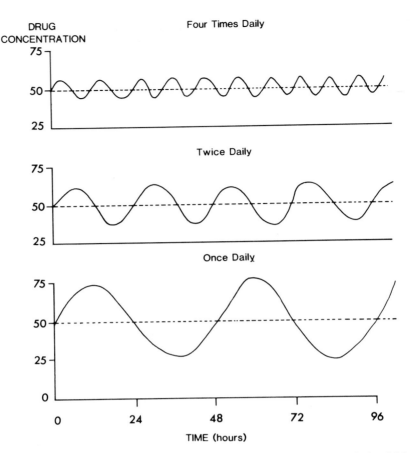

Fig. 1.10 Concentration-time curves at steady-state for a drug with a half-life of 24 hours given chronically in the same daily dose but divided into one, two or four increments. The steady-state (average) concentration is the same, namely 50 units, but with once daily dosage there is substantial hourly variation in concentration with high peaks and low troughs. This may be a drawback if side-effects relate closely to concentration, e.g. theophylline, carbamazepine. These drugs may better be given as a slow-release preparation (theophylline) or in divided doses (carbamazepine)

Pharmaceutics

Pharmaceutics is the science of drug design and formulation. The active agent's physicochemical characteristics such as lipid-water solubility, molecular weight and pH must be taken into consideration when a product is produced. The drug must be stable and bioavailable. Consistency of bioavailability is often more important than the percentage absorbed. Slow release formulations should be properly compared, both pharmacokinetically and pharmacodynamically, with a similar dose given as the original drug. Toxicity may also differ with a new formulation as occurred with osmotically-released indomethacin which produced an unacceptable incidence of small bowel ulceration and perforation. Novel routes of administration such as topical nitrates must produce satisfactory plasma levels as often as with the equivalent oral preparation. Patient acceptability is also an important factor. A bitter syrup of an antibiotic is unlikely to be palatable to an ill child. Consideration of the formulation may be an important factor in the choice of a therapeutic agent.

Pharmacodynamics

Pharmacodynamics is concerned with the relationship between drug concentration and effect with particular relevance to the time course of that effect, i.e. 'what the drug does to the patient'.

Pharmacogenetics

The control of drug metabolism represents a balance between genetic and environmental factors. There are two distinct genetic polymorphisms which may predispose to alterations in the response to and toxicity from certain drugs. The first of these involves acetylation of drugs such as hydralazine, isoniazid, phenelzine, procainamide, dapsone, nitrazepam and some sulphonamides. In the UK 45% of the population are slow acetylators and the rest rapid acetylators. Interestingly, there are considerable racial differences in the prevalence of the slow acetylator phenotype ranging from 22% in Eskimos to 91% in Egyptians. The half-lives of acetylated drugs are longer in slow than in fast acetylators. Thus, the former show a greater hypotensive response to hydralazine but are also more likely to develop a lupus-like syndrome with the drug. Side-effects with these drugs are in the main more common in slow acetylators. More recently a polymorphism affecting drug oxidation has also been described. About 9% of the population of the UK show reduced oxidative capacity for a number of drugs including debrisoquine, phenformin, nortriptyline, metoprolol and perhexiline. As a result poor oxidisers may be at greater risk of peripheral neuropathy with perhexiline or lactic acidosis with phenformin. The full clinical relevance of this oxidative polymorphism remains to be determined.

Pharmacokinetics

Pharmacokinetics is concerned with the study of the time course of drug absorption, distribution, metabolism and excretion with the aim of relating these to the therapeutic and adverse effects of drugs. It can be loosely described as 'what the patient does to the drug'. The kinetics and dynamics of a drug are interconnected, with the former responsible for the production of a given plasma or tissue concentration and the latter with the pharmacological or toxicological effect produced by that concentration (Fig. 1.11).

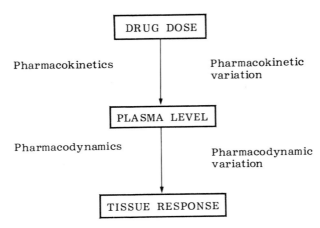

Fig.1.11 Relationship between the dose of a drug, its plasma level and the tissue response. There will be both pharmacokinetic and pharmacodynamic variation between patients

Predictable adverse effects

Most adverse effects of a drug are predictable from its pharmacological properties. These are sometimes called type A reactions and are usually dose-dependent. They occur by pharmaceutical, pharmacokinetic or pharmacodynamic mechanisms and will develop in all patients given a sufficiently large dose. Examples include heart block with digoxin, hypoglycaemia with glibenclamide and ataxia with phenytoin. This sort of adverse effect rarely causes a fatal reaction but is responsible for substantial morbidity. A reduction in dose will often be all that is necessary to ameliorate the problem.

Potency and efficacy

The potency of a drug is defined by its position along the horizontal axis of its dose-response curve (Fig. 1.5). Thus, the more potent the drug the lower the dose required to produce its pharmacological effect. The efficacy of a drug is the size of the response it produces. Potency differences can be overcome by giving an increased dose but maximal efficacy cannot be improved upon. This is illustrated in Fig. 1.12. Bendrofluazide (drug A) is a more potent diuretic than frusemide (drug B) since it is effective at a lower dose, but frusemide is more efficacious since it produces a greater diuresis. As an antihypertensive, however, bendrofluazide is more potent *and* more efficacious. In clinical practice, therefore, potency has little relevance.

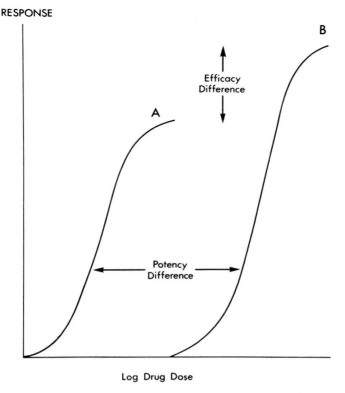

Fig. 1.12 Log dose response curves for drugs A and B. A (e.g. bendrofluazide) is more potent than B but B (e.g. frusemide) is more efficacious than A as a diuretic

Protein binding

Acidic and neutral drugs bind to albumin while basic drugs bind to globulins and acute phase reactants such as alpha$_1$ acid glycoprotein. Binding is rarely clinically relevant and only important if more than 90% of circulating drug is bound to plasma proteins. In chronic dosing, unbound (free) drug is responsible for its pharmacological and toxic effects (Fig. 1.13). If protein binding is reduced by disease or another competing drug, more free drug is available for metabolism and excretion and a similar steady-state unbound concentration is attained to that occurring if protein binding were normal. However, higher peak and lower trough concentrations are found and there is a compensatory fall in total drug concentration. Hence the extent and duration of the pharmacological effect may be subtly altered. Protein binding of acidic drugs such as warfarin and diazepam are reduced in disease states where serum albumin is low, e.g. cirrhosis, congestive cardiac failure, uraemia, third trimester of pregnancy. The binding of basic drugs such as propranolol and disopyramide may be increased in acute inflammatory conditions such as rheumatoid arthritis, Crohn's disease and following myocardial infarction. Protein binding

21

Pharmacological Glossary

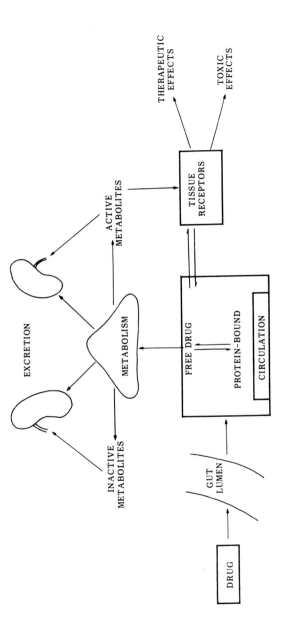

Fig. 1.13 Relationship between bound and free drug. Bound drug is trapped in the vascular space whereas unbound (free) drug is distributed throughout the tissues and is responsible for the pharmacological and toxic effects of the drug. The higher the amount unbound the greater its hepatic metabolism or renal excretion (first order kinetics). Therefore, when protein binding is reduced, steady-state free concentration is not increased but there is a compensatory fall in total plasma level

displacement interactions are rarely important on their own. If another mechanism is also operative such as inhibition of warfarin metabolism by phenylbutazone, an important adverse pharmacological event may ensue — in this case potentiation of anticoagulation. Changes in drug protein binding rarely influence prescribing although they may be responsible for increased susceptibility to toxic effects.

Receptors

Most drugs depend for their pharmacological (and toxic) effects on binding to a receptor of one kind or another. A receptor can be thought of as a specific tissue protein capable of binding drugs and endogenous substances. For most receptors there is a naturally occurring substance which binds to the receptor to trigger an appropriate biological response — an agonist. An antagonist is a chemical moiety, usually an exogenously administered drug, which blocks the effect of an agonist. The presence of a number of subtypes for each receptor allows drugs to be developed which have more specific pharmacological effects. Examples of these are shown in Table 1.4. This selectivity for a specific sub-type of receptor, e.g.

Table 1.4 Examples of drugs which depend on binding to receptors for their clinical effects

Receptor	Agonist	Antagonist
Cholinoreceptor	Carbachol	Atropine
	Bethanechol	Orphehadrine
		Pirenzepine
Adrenoceptors	Dobutamine (β_1)	Labetolol (α/β)
	Clonidine (α_2)	Prazosin (α_1)
	Salbutamol (β_2)	Atenolol (β_1)
		Propranolol (β_1/β_2)
Dopamine receptors	Bromocriptine	Chlorpromazine
		Haloperidol
		Metoclopramide
Histamine receptors	—	Promethazine (H_1)
		Cimetidine (H_2)
Opioid receptors	Morphine	Naloxone
	Buprenorphine	
Serotonin receptors	—	Ketotifen
		Cyproheptadine
GABA receptors	Baclofen	—
	Diazepam	

atenolol for β_1 receptors, is dose-dependent and so in high dosage atenolol can produce bronchospasm in a susceptible patient. Some drugs act as partial agonists (e.g. buprenorphine for opioid receptors) or partial antagonists (e.g. oxprenolol for β receptors). This may modify the side-effects of the drug so that they differ slightly from the pure agonist or antagonist. Thus, buprenorphine is relatively non-addictive because at high doses it also has antagonist properties; however it is also less effective as an analgesic than morphine. Similarly, because of its partial β agonist effect, oxprenolol causes less bradycardia than propranolol. This may be beneficial in patients with conduction defects or in the elderly, but is detrimental to the patient with thyrotoxicosis where the reduction in heart rate is an important therapeutic requirement. Because of the increasing knowledge of receptor pharmacology, it is now possible to design drugs to bind at a particular receptor prior to screening in the clinical setting. These advances will undoubtedly result in a flood of new, more specific therapeutic agents over the next decade.

Renal excretion

The excretion of drugs and their metabolites is largely carried out by renal glomerular and tubular mechanisms (Fig. 1.14). After

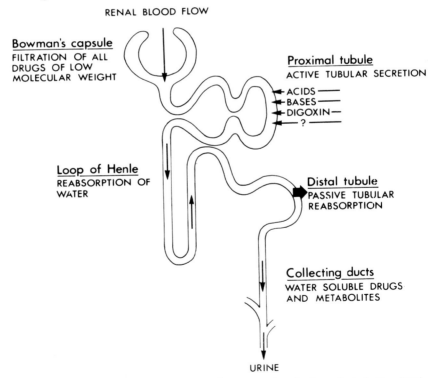

RENAL BLOOD FLOW

Bowman's capsule
FILTRATION OF ALL
DRUGS OF LOW
MOLECULAR WEIGHT

Proximal tubule
ACTIVE TUBULAR SECRETION
ACIDS ——
BASES ——
DIGOXIN —
— ? ——

Loop of Henle
REABSORPTION OF
WATER

Distal tubule
PASSIVE TUBULAR
REABSORPTION

Collecting ducts
WATER SOLUBLE DRUGS
AND METABOLITES

URINE

Fig. 1.14 All unbound drugs and metabolites are reabsorbed passively in the distal tubule and water soluble drugs and metabolites are eliminated in the urine. Some drugs are also actively secreted into the proximal tubule, and this mechanism may contribute substantially to their elimination, e.g. digoxin

glomerular filtration, lipid soluble drugs and metabolites passively diffuse back into the tubular cells and re-enter the circulation, whereas water soluble drugs and metabolites are eliminated directly in the urine. The renal tubular system can also actively secrete drugs. There are separate systems for the secretion of weak acids such as penicillins and cephalosporins and weak bases such as amiloride and ethambutol. Competition can occur between drugs using these transport mechanisms (Table 1.5). There is also a distinct secretory component for digoxin. Relatively few substances depend on renal excretion alone for elimination without prior oxidation or conjugation in the liver. For these water-soluble drugs clearance is dependent on glomerular filtration rate. If the drug has a narrow therapeutic ratio, e.g. lithium or digoxin, dosage must be adjusted in relation to impairment of renal function which is most conveniently measured as creatinine clearance.

Table 1.5 Acidic and basic drugs secreted actively by the kidney

Acids	Bases
Bumetanide	Amiloride
Cephalosporins	Cimetidine
Chlorpropamide	Ethambutol
Frusemide	Mepacrine
Indomethacin	Procainamide
Methotrexate	Ranitidine
Penicillins	
Phenobarbitone	
Phenylbutazone	
Probenecid	
Salicyclates	
Sulphonamides	
Thiazide diuretics	

Saturation kinetics

For most drugs in clinical use, first order kinetics apply, i.e. the rate of elimination from the body is directly proportional to the circulating concentration. For a few, the capacity for removal can be saturated and further drug is subject to zero order kinetics (Fig. 1.15). This is an important principle which may explain unexpected toxicity in a number of clinical settings. The best known examples involve drugs which have saturable hepatic metabolism such as phenytoin and ethanol. When saturation takes place a modest increment in dose can

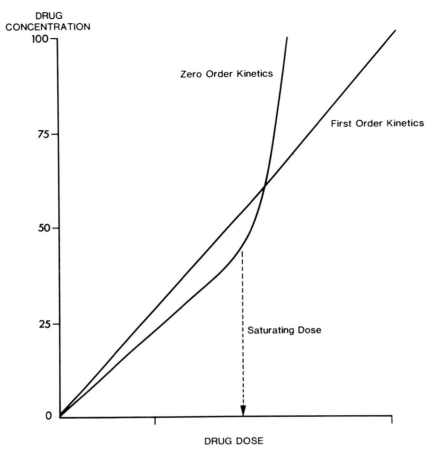

Fig. 1.15 Effect of increasing dose on concentration of drugs undergoing first order and saturation (zero order) kinetics. When saturation takes place, e.g. with phenytoin a further small increase in drug dose is reflected by a substantial rise in plasma concentration

result in a disproportionately large increase in drug level producing sudden toxicity. A clinical example is illustrated in Fig. 1.16.

Slow release preparations

There are many new long acting formulations of established drugs. These are designed to 'smooth out' the peak and trough concentrations and maintain a similar steady state level throughout the 24 hours. Some preparations are more successful than others. A short acting drug with a narrow therapeutic ratio and a clear concentration–effect relationship such as theophylline is ideal. Drugs with a half-life greater than 24 hours, e.g. diazepam or amitriptyline, are not appropriate for this type of formulation.

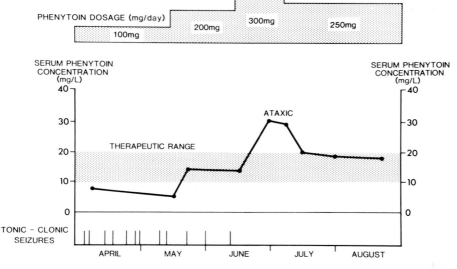

Fig. 1.16 Effect of increasing phenytoin dosage on seizure frequency and serum phenytoin concentration in a 75-year-old man with generalised tonic-clonic epilepsy following a cerebrovascular accident. On increasing the phenytoin dosage from 200 mg to 300 mg daily, plasma concentration trebled and overt signs of ataxia were apparent. On reducing the dose by only 50 mg, phenytoin concentration re-entered the therapeutic range and seizure control was maintained without side-effects.

Steady-state

When a number of drug doses are given over a period of time, the situation soon arises where the amount of drug absorbed is similar to that eliminated from the body, i.e. equilibrium or 'steady-state' has been reached (Fig. 1.17). The time taken for a drug to attain steady-state is mathematically a function of its half-life. Thus after one half-life 50% of steady-state is achieved; after two half-lives, 75%; after three, 87.5% and so on. For practical purposes, steady-state is obtained after five drug half-lives. This can be under 24 hours for a drug with a short half-life like morphine, or up to 10 days for digoxin, which has a half-life of 24–48 hours in a patient with normal renal function. If the concentration of the drug is closely related to its pharmacological effect, knowledge of its half-life is clearly clinically useful as for morphine, theophylline and phenytoin. For these drugs the half-life will allow prediction of the approximate time to maximum effect both on initiating therapy and changing doses. Similarly the rate of decay in response may be anticipated when the drug is discontinued. For other drugs such as prednisolone, propranolol and diazepam, where the pharmacodynamic effect does not readily relate to circulating concentration, knowledge of the half-life is less valuable.

27

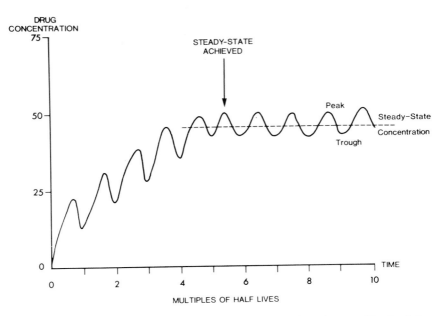

Fig. 1.17 Concentration-time curve on initiating chronic drug therapy. Steady-state concentration is reached after about five half-lives. The height of the peaks and depth of the troughs depends on the length of the half-life and the number of daily doses given

Subcutaneous injection

Bioavailability of drugs given subcutaneously depends on blood flow through the skin. In most instances, distribution is less variable than following intramuscular injection and subcutaneous injection may be a neglected route of drug administration. Currently insulin and heparin are the drugs most commonly administered subcutaneously. Beta agonists such as terbutaline can be given this way in severe asthma.

Sublingual preparations

A few lipid-soluble drugs are rapidly absorbed from the buccal mucosa producing a high, usually short-lived, plasma concentration within minutes, e.g. glyceryl trinitrate, nifedipine. Other longer-acting drugs such as buprenorphine may be administered by this route to avoid extensive first pass metabolism.

Suppositories

Rectal administration may prolong the duration of action of a drug and by-pass first pass metabolism to an extent. However, suppositories may cause local irritation, e.g. indomethacin and absorption is often erratic as with theophylline. Bioavailability tends to be lower than by the oral route. In some situations suppositories may be helpful such as oxycodone pectinate at night in terminal cancer. Generally, suppositories have no advantage over orally administered slow release preparations, e.g. theophylline and indomethacin.

Synergism

Drugs acting on the same system, organ, cell or enzyme may have synergistic properties. This may be clinically advantageous as with the components of the oral contraceptive pill or of co-trimoxazole. More often these drugs potentiate one another's adverse effects. Thus, all non-steroidal anti-inflammatory agents reduce platelet adhesiveness and will indirectly potentiate warfarin anticoagulation. From a knowledge of the pharmacology of the individual drugs these effects can be predicted. Hence calcium antagonists and beta-blockers, both of which have negative inotropic actions, may in combination precipitate cardiac failure in a susceptible patient.

Therapeutic range

The therapeutic range of a drug is a general guide to the circulating concentration expected to produce a pharmacological effect and that resulting in toxicity. It is based on data from a population of patients and may not be applicable to the individual. Thus, if a patient's seizure frequency is unaltered by increasing doses of phenytoin to the point of toxicity, a 'therapeutic range' of that drug for that patient does not exist. Similarly, epilepsy in another patient may be fully controlled with circulating phenytoin concentration of 5 mg/l which is lower than the accepted therapeutic range of 10–20 mg/l. Some patients can tolerate a phenytoin concentration far in excess of 20mg/l with clear-cut clinical benefit. The therapeutic range is best regarded as a target concentration band around which to adjust the dose of a drug according to clinical response or the development of side-effects.

Therapeutic ratio

The therapeutic ratio or index of a drug depends on the closeness of the relationship between the doses (and circulating concentrations) producing pharmacological and toxic effects. If the difference between these is wide, e.g. ampicillin or atenolol, the drug can be safely used in the majority of patients over a number of dosage increments. Drugs with a narrow therapeutic ratio, e.g. digoxin or phenytoin, have to be prescribed with more care and are much more likely to be implicated in adverse effects or interactions. Therapeutic drug monitoring may be employed to tailor the effective dose and avoid toxicity, e.g. for phenytoin, when an obvious pharmacological effect against which to titrate response is not available, e.g. prothrombin time with warfarin.

Tolerance

When an agonist drug is given chronically the number of receptor sites to which it can bind falls, i.e. 'down regulation' occurs. This may result in tolerance to its pharmacological effects. Tolerance to opiate analgesics may be a consequence of decreased numbers of opioid receptors. Similarly, athletes have reduced numbers of beta receptors on lymphocytes which may be the result of the high circulating levels of adrenaline and noradrenaline occurring during heavy training and in a race. This may, in part at least, explain their low resting pulse rate.

Topical preparations

Topical preparations may be used as slow-release formulations of rapidly metabolised drugs such as glyceryl trinitrate. Absorption from current formulations is variable and this route has no obvious advantage over oral long-acting nitrates. Topical formulations of some drugs may have the, as yet theoretical, advantage of avoiding first pass metabolism.

Water soluble drugs

Water soluble drugs are in the minority and are largely excreted unchanged by the kidney (Table 1.6). They are slowly and often incompletely absorbed. These drugs are less likely to cross the blood brain barrier in substantial amounts. Thus, atenolol can be substituted when propranolol produces vivid dreams or insomnia. They will cross the placenta and breast epithelium, although more slowly than lipid soluble drugs. Dosage reduction is normally required if renal function is impaired in proportion to the fall in glomerular filtration rate.

Table 1.6 Drugs excreted largely unchanged by the kidney

Acetohexamide	Digoxin
Acyclovir	Ethambutol
Amantadine	Flucytosine
Aminoglycosides	Frusemide
Atenolol	Guanethidine
Baclofen	Hyoscine
Bethanidine	Lithium
Bleomycin	Metformin
Bretylium	Methotrexate
Bumetanide	Nadolol
Cephalosporins	Penicillins
Chloroquine	Pirenzepine
Chlorothiazide	Procainamide
Chlorpropamide	Ranitidine
Cimetidine	Sotalol
Cisplatin	Tetracycline

Pharmacological Glossary

2

Drugs of Choice for Common Complaints

2

DECISION MAKING

In a number of clinical situations symptomatic drug therapy is employed. In others a curative approach is essential. In most instances a number of preparations and formulations are available. There is little comparative information to allow the prescriber to choose the most appropriate drug for the individual patient. Indeed the pharmaceutical industry representative remains the primary source of information for more than 60% of drugs which are actively promoted.

In this section our own 'best buy' drugs and preparations are outlined. Each decision takes efficacy, safety, convenience and cost into consideration and the rationale for each choice is briefly summarised. Most tables include a reserve drug and appropriate formulations. The relative cost is incorporated using the system employed in the British National Formulary with only minor modification. This is based on the price band for a week's course of treatment at the lowest dose stated, i.e.

A =   <20 p
B =   21–50 p
C =   51–100 p
D =   101–180 p
E =   181–300 p
F =   301–450 p
G =   >450 p

In the final column, the appropriate initial dose or dosage range is included. Throughout the book the approved (generic) drug names are used except for specific fixed drug combinations, e.g. Lomotil. The decision to prescribe has been assumed and this is not discussed in detail.

Clearly the drugs chosen are not the only effective agents available in each category or for each condition. They may not even be appropriate for all patients. However this approach does assume a decision-making process prior to each prescription. The prescriber must decide for himself whether to endorse our own choice or to consider which drug he would prefer to use and for what reason. This, of course, assumes some knowledge of the pharmacology and toxicology of the alternatives. Such therapeutic decision-making can readily be incorporated into the routine prescribing audit of a practice. The general practitioner may expect large rewards in improved patient care, professional satisfaction and financial savings from spending a little time reviewing his prescribing habits.

hoice	Preparation	Rationale	Cost	Dose
ntiseptic	Medicated soap	Cleansing Mild antiseptic	Price B	Substitute for conventional soap
opical	Benzoyl peroxide and sulphur cream (Benoxyl 5 with sulphur)	Keratolytic Cheapest	Price C	At night rub skin with hot damp flannel and apply cream
ystemic	Oxytetracycline 250 mg tablet	Well established Cheap	Price A	250 mg 12 hourly
	Avoid topical corticosteroids			

llergic conjunctivitis

hoice	Preparation	Rationale	Cost	Dose
orticosteroid	Prednisolone sodium phosphate 0.05% eye drops	Anti-inflammatory Intermittent use only	Price D	One drop instilled into each eye 4 hourly
ntihistamine	Antazoline 0.5% with xylometazoline 0.05% eye drops	Symptomatic relief	Price C	Two drops instilled into each eye 3 times a day
romoglycate	Sodium cromoglycate 2% eyedrops	Prophylaxis Long-term use	Price F	One drop instilled into each eye 4 times a day

llergic rhinitis

hoice	Preparation	Rationale	Cost	Dose
cute episode	Beclomethasone dipropionate nasal spray	Anti-inflammatory Effective Local effect	Price D	One 50 μg 'puff' into each nostril, up to four times a day
rophylaxis st choice	Sodium cromoglycate nasal spray	Local action Pharmacologically precise	Price G	One 2.6 mg 'puff' into each nostril six times a day
nd choice	Chlorpheniramine 12 mg tablet	Well tried Inexpensive Sedative	Price B	12 mg 12 hourly
	Terfenadine 60 mg tablet	Less sedative More expensive	Price D	60 mg 12 hourly

Drugs of Choice for Common Complaints

2

Analgesics

Choice	Preparation	Rationale	Cost	Dose
Mild pain				
1st choice	Paracetamol 500 mg tablet	Effective Few side-effects Cheap	Price A	0.5–1 g every 4–6 hours
2nd choice	Aspirin 300 mg effervescent tablet	Effective Cheap	Price B	600–900 mg every 4–6 hours dissolved in water
Moderate pain				
1st choice	Buprenorphine 200 μg sublingual tablet	Effective Partial opiate agonist	Price C	200–400 μg 4–6 hourly Sublingually
2nd choice	Naproxen 250 mg tablet	Anti-inflammatory Twice daily dose	Price E	250–750 mg every 12 hours
Severe pain				
1st choice	Morphine in aqueous solution 5–100 mg/10 ml in chloroform water	Effective Flexible formulation	Price C	5–100 mg every 4 hours
2nd choice	Morphine slow release (MST Continus) 10 mg, 30 mg, 60 mg tablets	Convenient preparation Less flexible	Price E	10–60 mg 2–3 times daily
Parenteral use	Diamorphine 5 mg, 10 mg, 30 mg ampoules	Rapid action Effective Use for immediate relief	Price C	5–10 i.v., i.m. or s.c. 4–6 hourly
Alternatives	Levorphanol 1.5 mg tablet	Less sedative Long acting	Price C	1.5–4.5 mg twice daily
	Phenazocine 5 mg tablet	Less sedative Less addictive	Price E	5–20 mg 4–6 hourly

Antacids

Choice	Preparation	Rationale	Cost	Dose
Suspensions 1st choice	Dijex	Magnesium/aluminium combination Cheapest	Price B	10 ml 4 hourly and at bedtime or as required
2nd choice	Sylopal	Also contains dimethicone	Price C	10 ml 4 hourly and at bedtime or as required
Tablets for use between liquid doses	Dijex	Magnesium/aluminium combination Cheapest	Price A	Chew 1–2 tablets as required

Antidepressants

Choice	Preparation	Rationale	Cost	Dose
1st choice	Imipramine 25 mg tablet	Effective Well established Less sedative Cheap	Price A	50–75 mg inititally as a single dose at bedtime
	Amitriptyline 25 mg tablet	Effective Well established Sedative Cheap	Price A	50–75 mg inititally as a single dose at bedtime
2nd choice	Mianserin 30 mg tablet	Fewer side-effects Sedative	Price D	30–60 mg initially as a single dose at bedtime
	Nomifensine 50 mg capsule	Fewer side-effects Less sedative Theoretical advantage in Parkinsonism	Price E	25–50 mg initially 2 or 3 times daily

Drugs of Choice for Common Complaints

Antidiarrhoeal drugs

Choice	Preparation	Rationale	Cost	Dose
1st choice	Kaolin mixture	Symptomatic treatment Safe Cheap	Price B	10–20 ml every 4 hours
2nd choice	Codeine phosphate 15 mg, 30 mg, 60 mg tablet	Effective Cheap	Price B	15–60 mg 3 times a day initially Avoid in infective diarrhoea
3rd choice	Loperamide 2 mg capsule	Effective Few side-effects	Price E	4 mg initially then 2 mg after each loose stool Avoid in infective diarrhoea

Antihistamines

Choice	Preparation	Rationale	Cost	Dose
1st choice	Chlorpheniramine 8 mg, 12 mg slow release formulation	Effective Cheap Twice daily dose	Price B	8–12 mg 12 hourly
2nd choice	Terfenadine 60 mg tablet	Less sedative	Price D	60 mg 12 hourly
	Astemizole 10 mg tablet	Less sedative Single daily dose	Price F	10 mg daily

Antipsychotics

Choice	Preparation	Rationale	Cost	Dose
1st choice	Chlorpromazine 25 mg, 50 mg, 100 mg tablets 25 mg/5 ml, 100 mg/5 ml syrups 10 mg/ml, 25 mg/ml injections	Well-tried Effective Cheap	Price A	25–100 mg tid according to response
2nd choice	Haloperidol 1.5 mg, 5 mg, 10 mg, 20 mg tablets 2 mg/ml elixir 5 mg/ml injection	Effective Useful if hyperactive Injection valuable for rapid control of severe behavioural disturbance	Price B	2.5–5 mg twice daily according to response 5–10 mg i.v. or i.m. for acute control of disturbed behaviour
Alternative	Pimozide 2 mg, 4 mg, 10 mg tablets	Used if apathetic or withdrawn Less sedative	Price F	4–10 mg nocte
	Thioridazine 10 mg, 25 mg, 50 mg, 100 mg tablets 25 mg/5 ml, 100 mg/5 ml suspensions 25 mg/5 ml syrup	Fewer extrapyramidal effects Used in elderly	Price B	25–100 mg tid according to response
Long-term therapy	Fluphenazine decanoate 12.5 mg, 25 mg, 50 mg ampoules 250 mg vial	Monthly injection Maintenance therapy	Price E	12.5 mg i.m. test dose (acute extrapyramidal symptoms) then 12.5–100 mg i.m. monthly according to response

Antitussives

Choice	Preparation	Rationale	Cost	Dose
First line	Steam inhalation	Sputum liquefaction	Nil	As required
	Simple linctus	Soothing placebo Useful in children	Price A	5 ml 4 times daily
	Methadone linctus 2 mg/5 ml	Effective for dry cough in terminal disease	Price B	5–10 ml 4–6 hourly
Second line	Codeine linctus 15 mg/5 ml	Dry cough Sometimes effective Constipating	Price B	5–10 ml 4 times daily

2

Drugs of Choice for Common Complaints

Anxiolytics

Choice	Preparation	Rationale	Cost	Dose
1st choice	Diazepam 2 mg, 5 mg, 10 mg tablets	Effective Long acting Cheap	Price A	2 mg–10 mg 3 times daily or at bedtime
If hepatic impairment	Lorazepam 1 mg, 2.5 mg tablets	Hepatic conjugation Use if liver disease	Price B	1–2.5 mg twice daily or at bedtime
If psychomotor impairment with other benzodiazepines	Clobazam 10 mg capsule	Less sedative	Price D	10 mg twice daily or at bedtime
In elderly	Thioridazine 25 mg/5 ml syrup	Sedative No tolerance	Price C	25 mg 2 or 3 times daily
Somatic symptoms	Propranolol 40 mg tablet	Blocks sympathetic overactivity Non-sedative	Price B	40 mg 2 or 3 times daily
	Intermittent use or short courses only			

Aphthous ulceration

Choice	Preparation	Rationale	Cost	Dose
First line	Soluble aspirin gargle	Analgesic Cheap	Price A	600 mg in water as a gargle 4 hourly
	Choline salicylate paste	Analgesic Local effect	Price C	Apply locally after meals and at bedtime
	Benzydamine oral rinse	Analgesic More expensive	Price E	15 ml 2 hourly or as required
	Carboxymethyl-cellulose gel	Local protection Expensive	Price E	Apply after meals Avoid hot drinks
Second line	Triamcinolone paste 0.1%	Corticosteroid Use if severe recurrent lesions	Price D	Apply sparingly after meals and at bedtime
	Tetracycline mouth bath	Antibiotic Use for severe lesions Avoid concurrent steroid	Price B	10 ml paediatric mixture held in the mouth for 3 minutes thrice daily
Third line	Low dose combined oral contraceptive	If associated with menstruation	Price B	One daily

Beta adrenoreceptor antagonists

Choice	Preparation	Rationale	Cost	Dose
Non-selective 1st choice	Propranolol 40 mg, 80 mg, 160 mg tablets	Well established Cheapest	Price C	40–320 mg 12 hourly
2nd choice	Nadolol 80 mg tablet	Long acting Excreted unchanged	Price G	80–240 mg daily
Cardioselective 1st choice	Atenolol 50 mg, 100 mg tablets	Single daily dose Water soluble Flat dose response	Price E	50–200 mg daily
Partial agonist activity 1st choice	Pindolol 5 mg, 15 mg tablets	Greatest partial agonism	Price E	5–15 mg 12 hourly

Cardioselective drug: Airways obstruction, intermittent claudication, cold extremities, insulin-dependent diabetes

Partial agonist drug: Bradycardia, potential cardiac failure, intermittent claudication, cold extremities

Water soluble drug: Depression, nightmares or insomnia with lipid soluble drug, hepatic cirrhosis

Corticosteroids

Choice	Preparation	Rationale	Cost	Dose
Topical	Hydrocortisone 1%, 2.5% cream/ointment (Efcortelan)	Potency IV (+)	Price B	Apply thinly to affected area up to 4 times daily
	Clobetasone butyrate 0.05% cream/ointment (Eumovate)	Potency III (+ +)	Price D	Apply thinly to affected area up to 4 times daily
	Betamethasone 0.1% cream/ointment (Betnovate)	Potency II (+ + +)	Price C	Apply thinly to affected area 1–2 times daily
	Clobetasol propionate 0.05% cream/ointment (Dermovate)	Potency I (+ + + +)	Price E	Apply thinly to affected area 1–2 times daily
Oral	Prednisolone 1 mg, 5 mg tablets	Effective Intermediate potency	Price A	5–80 mg daily according to indication
Intravenous	Hydrocortisone sodium succinate 100 mg, 500 mg vials	Effective Cheap	Price C	100–500 i.m. or i.v. according to indication

Diuretics

Choice	Preparation	Rationale	Cost	Dose
Thiazide diuretic	Bendrofluazide 2.5 mg, 5 mg tablets	Well established Cheap	Price A	2.5–10 mg daily
Loop diuretic	Frusemide 40 mg, 500 mg tablets 20 mg, 50 mg, 250 mg ampoules	Effective Cheap	Price B	40–250 mg once or twice daily 20–250 mg i.v. for immediate effect
Potassium-sparing diuretic	Amiloride 5 mg tablet	Effective Safe	Price D	5–20 mg daily

Dysmenorrhoea

Choice	Preparation	Rationale	Cost	Dose
1st choice	Ibuprofen 200 mg, 400 mg, 600 mg tablets	Prostaglandin inhibitor Few side-effects Over counter preparation	Price B	200–400 mg thrice daily
2nd choice	Naproxen 250 mg, 500 mg tablets	Prostaglandin inhibitor Greater efficacy Twice daily dosage	Price E	250–500 mg twice daily
Alternative	Mefenamic acid 500 mg tablet	Prostaglandin inhibitor Effective but higher incidence of side-effects	Price D	500 mg thrice daily
Persistent symptoms	Microgynon 30 or Ovranette	Inhibition of ovulation Balanced formulation	Price B	Ethinyloestradiol 30 μg Levonorgestrel 150 μg

Eczema

Choice	Preparation	Rationale	Cost	Dose
Soap substitute	Emulsifying ointment	Effective Cheap	Price A	As replacement for conventional soap
Emollient	Compound calamine application	Soothing Facilitates healing	Price A	Use for dry, fissured, scaly lesions
Astringent	Potassium permanganate 0.1%	Weeping lesions	Price A	Apply as wet dressing
Keratolytic	Coal tar and salicylic acid ointment	Chronic scaling Marked thickening	Price A	Apply once or twice daily
Topical steroid	Hydrocortisone 1%, 2.5% ointment	Effective Mild	Price B	Apply thinly up to 4 times daily

Drugs of Choice for Common Complaints

Glaucoma

Choice	Preparation	Rationale	Cost	Dose
1st choice	Timolol drops 0.25%, 0.5%	Beta blocker Twice daily dosage	Price G	Instil 1 or 2 drops twice daily
2nd choice	Pilocarpine drops 0.5, 1, 2, 3 and 4%	Miotic Cheap	Price B	Apply 3–6 times daily

Haematinics

Choice	Preparation	Rationale	Cost	Dose
Iron				
1st choice	Ferrous sulphate 300 mg tablet	Cheapest	Price A	300 mg 12 hourly with food
2nd choice	Ferrous fumarate 304 mg tablet	Fewer side-effects Single daily dose	Price B	Once daily with food
	Ferrous fumarate 140 mg/5 ml	Syrup	Price D	10 ml daily with food
In pregnancy	Ferrous fumarate and folic acid (Pregaday)	Combined iron and folate preparation	Price B	One daily with food (calendar pack)
Folic acid	Folic acid 5 mg tablet	Established folate deficiency	Price A	5 mg daily (prophylaxis) 5 mg tid (deficiency)
Vitamin B$_{12}$	Hydroxycobalamin 1 mg injection	Pernicious anaemia	Price A	1 mg i.m. weekly for 5 weeks (on diagnosis) 1 mg i.m. every 3 months (maintenance)

Hypnotics

Choice	Preparation	Rationale	Cost	Dose
1st choice	Temazepam 10 mg, 20 mg capsules	Effective Short half-life	Price C	10–20 mg 30 minutes before bedtime
2nd choice	Triazolam 125, 250 μg tablets	Effective Short half-life	Price C	125–250 μg 30 minutes before bedtime
Elderly	Chlormethiazole syrup 500 mg/10 ml	Syrup formulation Sedative No hangover	Price C	10 ml in water 30 minutes before bedtime
Children	Promethazine elixir 5 mg/5 ml	Elixir preparation Sedative No dependence	Price B	5–25 ml 30 minutes before bedtime
		Intermittent use only		

Infection: abdominal

Choice	Preparation	Rationale	Cost	Dose
Pelvic inflammation	Doxycycline 100 mg capsule Metronidazole 400 mg tablets	Active against anaerobes, chlamydia and mycoplasma Synergistic	Price G Price F	100 mg twice daily for 10 days 400 mg twice daily for 10 days
Chronic appendicitis	Amoxycillin 250 mg capsule Metronidazole 400 mg tablet	Active against aerobes and anaerobes Synergistic	Price F Price F	250 mg thrice daily for 5 days 400 mg thrice daily for 5 days
Cholecystitis	Cephradine 500 mg capsule	Safe Effective Good biliary penetration	Price G	500 mg 4 times daily for 7–10 days

Infection: ENT

Choice	Preparation	Rationale	Cost	Dose
Tonsillitis	Penicillin V 250 mg capsule 125 mg/5 ml syrup	Effective Cheap	Price B Price D	250 mg 4 times daily before food for 5 days 125 mg 3 times daily before food for 5 days (child under 10)
Sinusitis	Erythromycin 250 mg, 500 mg tablets	Effective Safe	Price C	250–500 mg 4 times daily for 5 days
Dental infection	Amoxycillin 250 mg capsule	Aerobic infection	Price F	250 mg 3 times daily as necessary
	Metronidazole 400 mg tablet	Anaerobic infection	Price F	400 mg 3 times daily as necessary
Otitis media	Penicillin V 250 mg tablet 125 mg/5 ml syrup	Adult and older child Child under 10	Price B Price D	250 mg 4 times daily before food for 5 days 125 mg 4 times daily before food for 5 days
	Amoxycillin 125 mg/5 ml syrup	Child under 5 May be haemophilus	Price D	125 mg 3 times daily for 5 days

fection: eye

hoice	Preparation	Rationale	Cost	Dose
epharitis	Propamidine isethionate 0.1% drops	Local effect Antibacterial	Price C	Apply 4 times daily
onjunctivitis	Chloramphenicol 0.5% drops 1% ointment	Broad-spectrum Effective	Price B Price C	Apply every 3 hours
endritic orneal cer	Acyclovir 3% ointment	Specific Effective Safe	Price G	Apply 5 times daily
achoma	Tetracycline 1% ointment	Cheap Effective	Price C	Apply 3 times daily for 6 weeks

fection: genito-urinary

hoice	Preparation	Rationale	Cost	Dose
st choice JTI)	Trimethoprim 200 mg tablet	Lower UTI Safe Effective	Price D	200 mg twice daily for 5 days
nd choice JTI)	Amoxycillin 3 g sachet	Uncomplicated UTI Convenient	Price F	1 sachet in water repeated after 12 hours
yelonephritis	Co-trimoxazole double strength 960 mg dispersible tablet	Effective	Price D	One tablet twice daily for 7 days. High fluid intake
aginal andidosis	Clotrimazole pessary	Convenient Cosmetically acceptable	Price E	One pessary inserted nightly for 3 nights
aginal ichomoniasis	Metronidazole 400 mg tablet	Effective Convenient	Price D	800 mg in the morning and 1200 mg at night for 2 days Treat consort
on-specific rethritis	Oxytetracycline 500 mg tablet	Exclude syphilis and gonorrhoea	Price A	500 mg thrice daily for 2–3 weeks

Drugs of Choice for Common Complaints

Infection: respiratory

Choice	Preparation	Rationale	Cost	Dose
1st choice	Amoxycillin 250 mg capsule 250 mg/5 ml syrup forte	Effective Well absorbed Well tolerated	Price F	250 mg 3 times daily for 5 days
2nd choice	Co-trimoxazole double strength 960 mg	Effective More side-effects	Price D	One tablet twice daily for 5 days
Chronic bronchitis	Oxytetracycline 250 mg, 500 mg tablets	Effective against *H. influenzae* Cheap	Price A	250–500 mg 4 times daily for 7 days
Penicillin-sensitivity	Erythromycin 250 mg, 500 mg tablets	Well tolerated Useful alternative	Price C	250–500 mg 4 times daily for 5 days

Infection: skin

Choice	Preparation	Rationale	Cost	Dose
1st choice	Flucloxacillin 250 mg capsule	Boils Impetigo Cellulitis	Price F	250 mg 4 times daily before meals
	Penicillin V 250 mg capsule	Erysipelas	Price B	250–500 mg 4 times daily before meals
2nd choice	Erythromycin 250 mg, 500 mg tablets	Penicillin allergy	Price C	250–500 mg 4 times daily
	Chlortetracycline 3% cream/ointment	Mild infection	Price E	Apply thrice daily
Ringworm	Griseofulvin 500 mg tablet *and*	Systemic	Price E	500 mg daily with meals for 4 weeks
	Clotrimazole 1% cream	Topical Use alone for athlete's foot	Price D	Apply twice daily for 4 weeks
Candidosis	Amphotericin 10 mg lozenge	Oral thrush	Price D	Dissolve 1 slowly in the mouth 4 times daily
	Clotrimazole 1% cream	Cutaneous lesions	Price D	Apply twice daily
Viral	Acyclovir 5% cream	Herpes simplex	Price G	Apply 5 times daily for 5 days

...hoice	Preparation	Rationale	Cost	Dose
...st choice	High roughage, high fluid diet	Natural	—	—
...d choice	Bran	Physiological	Non-prescription	4–6 heaped 5–8 ml spoonfuls daily mixed with food High fluid intake
...d choice	Sterculia with frangula (Normacol standard)	Easier tolerated Bulk former	Price C	1–2 heaped 5 ml spoonfuls once or twice daily after main meal or at bedtime
...inful anal ...sions	Liquid paraffin and magnesium hydroxide mixture	Faecal softener	Price A	10–20 ml every 12 hours
...patic failure	Lactulose elixir	Osmotic effect	Price C	30–50 ml thrice daily

...ausea

...hoice	Preparation	Rationale	Cost	Dose
...eneral ...astro-...testinal ...sease	Metoclopramide 10 mg tablets 5 mg/5 ml elixir 10 mg/2 ml injection	Central and local effects Non-sedative	Price C	10–20 mg three times daily
...byrinthine ...sorders, ...aemia, ...oplasia, ...st-radiation	Prochlorperazine 5 mg, 25 mg tablets 5 mg/5 ml syrup 12.5 mg/ml injection	Central effect Sedative	Price B	10–25 mg initially then 10 mg 2 hours later if necessary and 5–10 mg thrice daily thereafter
...ecialised ...otion ...ckness	Hyoscine hydrobromide 0.3 mg, 0.6 mg tablets	Effective Cheap	Price A or over the counter	0.3–0.6 mg 30 minutes before journey and up to four times daily thereafter
...orning ...ckness of ...egnancy	Promethazine theoclate 25 mg tablet	Effective Safe	Price A	25 mg–75 mg at bedtime
...evention of ...totoxic ...duced ...nesis	Nabilone 1 mg tablet	Cannabinoid Specific central effect	Price J (hospital only)	1–2 mg twice daily throughout each treatment cycle

2

Drugs of Choice for Common Complaints

Non-steroidal anti-inflammatory agents

Choice	Preparation	Rationale	Cost	Dose
1st choice	Ibuprofen 200 mg, 400 mg, 600 mg tablets	Few side-effects Cheap	Price B	200–600 mg 3 or 4 times daily
	Naproxen 250 mg, 500 mg tablets	Greater efficacy Twice daily dosage	Price E	250–750 mg twice daily
Alternatives	Piroxicam 10 mg capsule	Effective Single daily dose	Price E	10–30 mg once daily
	Indomethacin 75 mg slow release capsule	Highly efficacious Useful for morning stiffness Side-effects common	Price D	75 mg at night or twice daily

All non-steroidal anti-inflammatory agents should be taken with food

Oral contraceptives

Choice	Preparation	Rationale	Cost	Dose
1st choice	Microgynon 30 or Ovranette	Balanced preparation	Price B	Ethinyloestradiol 30 μg Levonorgestrel 150 μg
	IF BREAKTHROUGH Norimin	Increased oestrogen and progestogen doses	Price C	Ethinyloestradiol 35 μg Norethisterone 1 mg
	IF STILL BREAKTHROUGH Minovlar	Increased oestrogen dose	Price B	Ethinyloestradiol 50 μg Norethisterone 1 mg
Triphasic preparation (less effective)	Logynon	Mimics normal hormonal cycle	Price C	Phased ethinyloestradiol and norethisterone in 3 dosages
Progestogen only (less effective)	Femulen	Fewer side-effects	Price C	Ethynodiol diacetate 500 μg

hoice	Preparation	Rationale	Cost	Dose
st choice	Aluminium acetate 13% ear drops	Astringent	Price A	Apply using a gauze wick 3 times daily
d choice	Betamethasone 0.1% drops	Steroid	Price C	Apply every 3 hours
cterial ection	Chloramphenicol 5% drops	Local effect Broad spectrum	Price C	Apply 3 times daily
il	Flucloxacillin 250 mg capsule	Specific for penicillin-resistent staphyloccoci	Price F	250 mg 4 times daily before food for 5 days

soriasis

hoice	Preparation	Rationale	Cost	Dose
mollient	Aqueous cream	Cosmetically acceptable Cheap	Price A	Use for mild lesions
oal tar	Zinc and coal tar paste	Antipruritic Keratolytic	Price A	Apply at night
	Carbo-Dome cream	Use on face	Price D	Apply twice daily
	Coal tar solution	Extensive lesions	Price C	Use in bath
thranol	Psoradrate cream 0.1%, 0.2%	Severe lesions Cosmetically acceptable	Price E	Apply twice daily after tar bath
hampoo	Polytar liquid	Scalp lesions Removal of pastes	Price E	Use twice weekly or as necessary
pical steroid	Hydrocortisone cream 1%, 2.5%	Flexural lesions only	Price B	Apply sparingly twice daily
	Avoid potent topical steroids			

Sex hormone replacement therapy

Choice	Preparation	Rationale	Cost	Dose
Testosterone	Restandol 40 mg capsule	Testosterone ester Oral preparation	Price G	40 mg 3 times daily initially, 40–80 mg maintenance dosage
Oestrogen with	Ethinyloestradiol 10 μg tablet	Cheap Effective Menopausal symptoms	Price A	10–20 μg daily
Progestogen	Norethisterone 5 mg tablet	Balance effect of oestrogen Menopausal symptoms	Price E	5 mg daily for days 17–26 of cycle
Combined	Prempak-C 0.625	Menopausal symptoms	Price F	One daily from calendar pack

Vestibular disorders

Choice	Preparation	Rationale	Cost	Dose
1st choice	Hyoscine hydrobromide 300 μg, 600 μg tablets	Very effective Cheap	Price A	300–600 μg 4 times daily
2nd choice	Cinnarizine 15 mg tablet	Fewer side effects	Price C	15–30 mg 3 times daily
	Prochlorperazine 5 mg tablet	Useful in acute attack or if vomiting	Price B	5 mg 3 times daily

Vitamin supplements

Choice	Preparation	Rationale	Cost	Dose
Deficiency (Rare)	Vitamins A and D capsules	Contains A 4000u ⎫ Contains D 400u ⎬	Price A	One daily (prophylaxis)
	Ro–A–Vit	Contains 50 000u	Price B	One daily (deficiency)
Deficiency	Vitamin B compound strong tablets	Contains nicotinamide pyridoxine, riboflavine, thiamine	Price A	One once or twice daily (prophylaxis) One or two thrice daily (deficiency)
Deficiency	Ascorbic acid 25 mg, 50 mg, 100 mg, 200 mg, 500 mg tablets	Effective Cheap	Price A	25–75 mg daily (prophylaxis) 200–500 mg twice daily (deficiency)
Deficiency	Vitamins A and D capsules	Contains D 400u Contains A 4000u ⎫ ⎬	Price A	One daily (prophylaxis)
	Calciferol high strength 250 µg tablets	Higher vitamin D content	Price B	250 µg–1 mg daily (deficiency)
Multivitamin deficiency, e.g. elderly, alcoholic, cirrhotic	Vitamins capsule	Contains A, B, C, D Cheapest	Price A	One daily (prophylaxis)

Drugs of Choice for Common Complaints

3

Drug Treatment
Policies

DRUG TREATMENT POLICIES

There are a number of common conditions for which drugs are the mainstay of management. These may be used singly but are often combined in an attempt to produce a synergistic response with the avoidance of toxicity. With the advent of new and more effective therapeutic agents, the wider choice of drugs may lead to inappropriate prescribing. This is particularly important as prescription of drugs for these conditions may be lifelong. In this section, drug treatment of a number of disease states is considered and a 'policy' approach is adopted. The assumption that drug therapy is appropriate has been made and the factors involved in this decision are not discussed. The regimens listed are not meant to be inflexible and can clearly be altered in the light of newer agents becoming available or individual knowledge and preference. Substitution of different drugs within the plan can readily be made. It is important to understand the clinical pharmacology of the chosen drugs. This approach is designed to reduce the number of drugs employed in the treatment of a particular condition and refine the use of the few well-established preparations chosen. All prescribers should have their own treatment policies based on knowledge of the pathophysiology of the disease, the clinical pharmacology of the available drugs and their own clinical experience.

ANGINA

The drug treatment of angina is aimed at reducing myocardial oxygen demand and increasing coronary artery blood flow. It is based on the use of nitrates in combination with beta blockers and/or calcium antagonists. The majority of patients have fixed stenosis of one or more coronary arteries and for these beta blockers are first line agents. A few have coronary artery spasm and here calcium antagonists are preferred. Occasionally beta blockers may exacerbate coronary arteriospasm.

First line

GLYCERYL TRINITRATE   0.5 mg sublingually p.r.n.

and

PROPRANOLOL   40–320 mg b.d.

or

ATENOLOL   50–200 mg daily
(underlying COAD, peripheral vascular disease, insulin-dependent diabetes)

or

VERAPAMIL   80–240 mg b.d.
(beta blocker contra-indicated or not tolerated, coronary artery spasm)

Second line GLYCERYL TRINITRATE/BETA BLOCKER

and

ISOSORBIDE
MONONITRATE   10–40 mg b.d.–t.i.d.

and/or

NIFEDIPINE   10–30 mg t.i.d.
(also immediate effect in coronary artery spasm by biting into capsule and retaining liquid in mouth)

N.B.   Combination of verapamil with a beta blocker should be avoided as they have additive effects in reducing myocardial contractility and slowing cardiac conduction.

ANAPHYLAXIS

Anaphylaxis or other severe allergic reactions such as angioneurotic oedema are initiated by allergic material reacting with antibodies fixed on cells, particularly mast cells and basophils This results in the release of pharmacological mediators such as histamine, serotonin, kinins and prostaglandins. The resultant reaction develops within minutes and manifests primarily as shock. Precipitating agents include insect stings, drugs such as penicillins, local anaesthetics, blood products, vaccines and radioopaques dyes (invasive radiological procedures). Treatment is aimed at pharmacological modification of the effects of the released vasoactive substances. The patient should first be laid flat and the feet elevated.

1. ADRENALINE (1:1000) 0.5–1 ml i.m.

    or

    ADRENALINE Min-i-Jet 0.5–1 ml i.m.

    and

2. HYDROCORTISONE HEMISUCCINATE 200 mg i.v.

    and

3. CHLORPHENIRAMINE 10 mg i.v. slowly
    If no response, repeat **1** immediately and again in 15 minutes.

4. If severe angioneurotic oedema, consider tracheal intubation.

5. If still shocked, DOBUTAMINE 5 μg/kg/min by intravenous infusion.

ASTHMA

The aim of treatment in this variable condition is to restore the calibre of the airways to normal and prevent further bronchospasm. All treatment should be monitored by serial objective measurement using a peak flow meter. Following a severe acute asthmatic attack, a number of pharmacological approaches may be combined and when bronchospasm has been eliminated oral therapy may be substituted by less toxic topical treatment via inhalers.

First line

1. β_2 ADRENOCEPTOR AGONISTS — cheapest
   TERBUTALINE

   (a) by inhalation p.r.n. — q.i.d., symptomatically and prophylactically.

   (b) By spacer q.i.d., if unable to coordinate inhaler

   (c) by nebuliser q.i.d., if severe acute attack

   (d) intravenously — acute asthma attack. Single dose prior to hospital admission. No more effective than by nebuliser but preferred to intravenous aminophylline as less toxic.

   (e) oral — confine to small children and few patients unable to use inhalers. Slow release preparations usually ineffective in nocturnal asthma.

2. SODIUM CROMOGLYCATE — Spincaps q.i.d.

   prophylaxis in children with allergic and exercise-induced asthma. Less effective in adults.

Second line

1. XANTHINES-NUELIN SA, THEO–DUR, PHYLLOCONTIN CONTINUS are best long-acting preparations, b.d. administration.
   Aim for circulating theophylline concentration > 10 mg/l. At high concentrations (usually > 20 mg/l) nausea, vomiting, headache, agitation and diarrhoea can occur and can be relieved by reducing the dose. Cardiac arrythmias and seizures if > 30 mg/l and hence i.v. aminophylline contraindicated if patient receiving oral theophylline.
   Large single dose at night may relieve nocturnal bronchospasm.

2.　　CORTICOSTEROIDS BY INHALATION — prophylactically

BECLOMETHASONE DIPROPIONATE　b.d. — q.i.d.

BETAMETHASONE VALERATE　　　b.d. — q.i.d.

BUDESONIDE　　　　　　　　　　b.d.

Patients unable to coordinate inhaler may benefit from dry powder insufflator or spacer. Used with β_2 agonist. Should not be taken p.r.n. as may take several weeks for maximal benefit.

3.　　IPRATROPIUM BROMIDE　b.d. — q.i.d., cholinergic antagonist
Used with β_2 agonist and theophylline. Most useful in chronic bronchitis and elderly asthmatics.
In severe cases nebulised ipratropium may be given in combination with a β_2 agonist.

Third line

1.　　CORTICOSTEROIDS BY MOUTH

PREDNISOLONE 30 mg daily for 5 days or until improvement in peak flow plateaus out. Single morning dose causes less adrenal suppression. Use with β_2 agonist and theophylline. Reduce dose slowly and introduce corticosteroid inhaler.
Few patients require to be maintained on prednisolone 7.5 mg/day or less.

2.　　CORTICOSTEROIDS INTRAVENOUSLY

HYDROCORTISONE 200–400 mg i.v. if life-threatening episode.
Administer prior to hospital admission.
Effects are delayed for 4–6 hours but probably speeds recovery and may be life-saving in severe asthma.

BELL'S PALSY

Treatment only indicated within a few days of onset of paresis.

PREDNISOLONE 10 mg q.i.d. for 7 days

then reduce and stop over the next 2 weeks

and

HYPROMELLOSE EYE DROPS ⎫
SUNGLASSES ⎬ if required
⎭

and

ASPIRIN OR PARACETAMOL for facial pain

CARDIAC FAILURE

As the population gets older, the prevalence of cardiac failure has increased. There has been a drift away from positive inotropic agents such as digoxin to the more logical policy of reducing cardiac pre-load and after-load with venous and arteriolar vasodilators. The use of potassium supplements both separately and combined with diuretics has been subject to criticism as larger amounts of potassium are needed than readily supplied by these preparations. Most patients receiving diuretics such as frusemide or bumetanide do not develop symptomatic hypokalaemia. If hypokalaemia < 3 mmol/l develops, the patient is symptomatic or taking concurrent digoxin, a potassium-sparing diuretic such as amiloride or spironolactone will oppose pharmacologically the potassium loss. Potassium-sparing diuretics should be avoided in patients with renal failure as hyperkalaemia may insidiously develop. Patients with renal failure do not normally develop hypokalaemia.

First line	FRUSEMIDE	40–120 mg daily or b.d.
		or
	BUMETANIDE	0.5 – 3 mg daily or b.d.
		and if hypokalaemia < 3 mmol/l or on digoxin
	AMILORIDE	5–20 mg daily
		or
	SPIRONOLACTONE	100–300 mg daily

Drug Treatment Policies

3

Second line	VASODILATORS	*add* 1, 2 or 3
1.	PRAZOSIN	0.5–5 mg t.i.d.–q.i.d. (arteriolar and venous vasodilator)
2.	HYDRALAZINE	25–100 mg b.d.–q.i.d. (arteriolar vasodilator — particularly if congestive failure)
3.	ISOSORBIDE DINITRATE	10–40 mg t.i.d.–q.i.d. (venous vasodilator — particularly if chronic left ventricular failure; can be combined with hydralazine)

and/or

Third line DIGOXIN 0.5–1 mg loading dose
0.0625–0.5 mg daily maintenance dose

If fast atrial fibrillation, use as first line drug
Maintenance dose depends on renal function as follows:

Daily digoxin dose (mg)	Creatinine clearance (ml/min)	Approximate serum creatinine (μmol/l)
0.5	80–120	75
0.25	50–80	100
0.1875	25–50	200
0.125	10–25	300
<0.0625	<10	>400

Lower dose if combined with quinidine, verapamil or amiodarone

Fourth line

CAPTOPRIL 12.5–50 mg b.d.
(venous and arteriolar vasodilator — in end stage cardiac failure)

First dose may cause hypotension. Start with 6.25 mg daily and increase slowly.

DIABETES MELLITUS

The aim of treatment in the insulin-dependent (type 1) diabetic is to maintain normoglycaemia for as much of the 24 hours of each day as possible to prevent the development of vascular complications. Since insulin secretion fluctuates from minute to minute, this is difficult to achieve for most diabetics even with three injections of insulin daily. Combinations of insulins of differing half-lives are employed and these are best determined on an individual basis, by gradually increasing the dose and monitoring plasma glucose concentrations throughout the day with BM stix or an Ames glucometer. The current insulins of choice are the highly purified insulins of animal origin. There is no obvious advantage in using the more expensive human insulins.

For the patient taking oral hypoglycaemic agents (type 2 diabetics) the more modest aim is to keep the urine free of glucose with the avoidance of hypoglycaemia. In the elderly a more cautious policy of keeping the patient symptom-free is acceptable as the symptoms of hypoglycaemia, especially nocturnal, can be insidious. Insulin may be required during intercurrent illness, e.g. myocardial infarction, infection and during surgery.

Diagnosis

> Plasma glucose <6 mmol/l — diabetes excluded
> Fasting plasma glucose >8 mmol/l — diabetes confirmed
> Random plasma glucose >11 mmol/l — diabetes confirmed

If fasting plasma glucose 6–8 mmol/l — do 75 g oral GTT
If 2 hour plasma glucose >11 mmol/l — diabetes confirmed
If 2 hour plasma glucose 8–11 mmol/l — 'impaired glucose tolerance'

Type 1: insulin dependent

DIET — FAT AND CARBOHYDRATE RESTRICTION

> **and**

> PURIFIED INSULIN s.c. — before breakfast and evening meal

First line

> ACTRAPID MC b.d.

> **and**

> SEMITARD MC b.d.

Second line

> ULTRATARD MC before evening meal

> **with/without**

> ACTRAPID MC before breakfast and lunch

Type 2: Non-insulin dependent

DIET — CALORIE, FAT and CARBOHYDRATE RESTRICTION

   with/without

First line

   GLIBENCLAMIDE 2.5–10 mg b.d.

   or

   GLIQUIDONE 15–60 mg daily — t.i.d. with meals
                  (younger patient, more precise control)

   and/or

Second line METFORMIN 0.5–1 g daily — t.i.d. with food
   (used alone in obese patients, small risk of lactic
   acidosis)

DYSPEPSIA

There are now a number of potent gastric antisecreting drugs available and these should not be used until a specific diagnosis has been made, particularly in the middle-aged or elderly patient.

Initial therapy — 4 weeks

(a)   ANTACIDS p.r.n. — liquids preferred
      Aluminium hydroxide — if tendency to diarrhoea
      Magnesium trisilicate — if tendency to constipation
      Sylopal (with dimethicone) — if also heartburn

(b)   Small frequent meals

(c)   Stop smoking

(d)   Reduce alcohol, tea and coffee consumption

      If symptoms still troublesome after *4 weeks* non-specific therapy then arrange barium meal

If DUODENAL ULCER
      Antacids p.r.n.

      and

First line   H$_2$ RECEPTOR ANTAGONIST

RANITIDINE 150 mg b.d.

(fewer adverse effects

and interactions)

or

CIMETIDINE 400 mg b.d.

} for 6–8 weeks, then single dose at night for further 3–6 months

or

Second line SUCRALFATE 1 g q.i.d. for 4–8 weeks — local action
(constipation major side-effect)

or

BISMUTH CHELATE 5 ml t.i.d. before meals and at
bedtime for 4–6 weeks — local action
(may blacken faeces)

or

Third line   PIRENZEPINE 50 mg b.d.–t.i.d. for 4–8 weeks —
muscarinic antagonist
(occasionally dry mouth, visual disturbance, urinary
difficulty)

or

CARBENOXOLONE SODIUM 50 mg q.i.d. for 6–12
weeks — increases mucus production
(hypokalaemia, oedema and hypertension can occur,
particularly in the elderly)

If GASTRIC ULCER — endoscopy and biopsy to
exclude carcinoma in middle-aged or elderly patients
(4% of gastric ulcers are malignant). Then, treat as for
duodenal ulcer. May require longer duration of therapy if
large ulcer.

If HIATUS HERNIA WITH OESOPHAGEAL REFLUX
Advice on posture, smoking, alcohol consumption and
diet

First line   MUCAINE or SYLOPAL p.r.n.

and/or

GAVISCON LIQUID 10–20 ml 30 minutes after meals
and at bedtime for 2 weeks

with/without

METOCLOPRAMIDE 10 mg t.i.d.

or

DOMPERIDONE 10–20 mg t.i.d.

Second line   RANITIDINE 150 mg b.d. ⎫
  or   ⎬ for 6 weeks
  CIMETIDINE 400 mg b.d. ⎭

  or

  SUCRALFATE 1 g q.i.d.   for 6 weeks

  or

Third line   Bethanechol 10 mg t.i.d. before food for 4 weeks
  (avoid in elderly patients)

  or

  PYROGASTRONE 1 tablet t.i.d. and 2 at bedtime
  (chewed) for 6–12 weeks
  (contains carbenoxolone)

If X-RAY NEGATIVE, then endoscope. If endoscopy and
  oral cholecystogram negative

  (a)   continue non-specific treatment

    with/without

  (b)   trial of H_2 antagonist

    or

  (c)   trial of sucralfate

EPILEPSY

As many epileptic patients recieve anticonvulsants life-long, consideration of the risk-benefit ratio for individual agents is of particular importance. There is no evidence that polytherapy is more effective than monotherapy. Epidemiological data suggest that poor control in the first year of the disease may condemn the patient to a lifetime of intermittent seizures and multiple anticonvulsants.

Consequently, optimum use of the most appropriate anti-epileptic agent, often with the help of therapeutic drug monitoring, early in the clinical course is essential. Treatment should begin with a first line agent, initially in low dosage with slow titration over 6 weeks to attain a plasma concentration well within the target range. In the early stages of treatment the daily dose should be divided as little as possible. If the patient is intolerant of the first drug, a second agent should be introduced and the first gradually withdrawn. Polytherapy should only be considered when all reasonable single drug options have been exhausted. Even with the best treatment only 70–80% of patients with generalised tonic clonic and around 50% with partial epilepsy will remain completely seizure-free.

Classification of epileptic seizures

(International League against Epilepsy, 1980)

GENERALISED SEIZURES — symmetrical

1. Absence seizures — 'Petit mal'
2. Tonic-clonic seizures — 'Grand mal'
3. Myoclonic seizures — 'Myoclonic jerks'
4. Tonic seizures ⎫
5. Akinetic seizures ⎭ Very rare

PARTIAL SEIZURES — focal

1. Simple — without impairment of consciousness ⎫ 'Focal' / 'Jacksonian'
2. Complex — with impairment of consciousness ⎬ 'Temporal lobe' / 'Psychomotor'

(A) Generalised tonic—clonic
('Grand mal')

First line SODIUM VALPROATE   200–600 mg b.d.–q.i.d.
10–30 mg/kg b.d. (child)
(small risk of hepatotoxicity, thrombocytopenia, pancreatitis)

or

CARBAMAZEPINE   100–400 mg b.d.–q.i.d.
50–200 mg b.d.–q.i.d. (child)
(start low dose to avoid sedation, nausea, headache, and build up as tolerance occurs; small risk of blood dyscrasia)

or

Second line PHENYTOIN   100–600 mg nocte
5–8 mg/kg/day (child)
(plasma level monitoring essential; cosmetic effects, teratogenicity; small risk of hepatotoxicity, blood dyscrasia, lymphoma)

and

Third line CLONAZEPAM   0.5–4 mg b.d.
0.125–3 mg daily (child)
(sedation invariable at higher doses)

or

PHENOBARBITONE   90–375 mg nocte or divided doses
5–10 mg/kg/day (child)
(never use alone except for febrile convulsions; withdrawal seizures a major problem)

or

CLOBAZAM   20–30 mg nocte or divided doses
10–15 mg nocte or divided doses
(children over 3 years)

Partial simple, complex or secondary generalised
('Focal', 'Temporal lobe', 'Jacksonian', 'Psychomotor')

First line   CARBAMAZEPINE

              or

Second line PHENYTOIN

              or

              SODIUM VALPROATE

              and

Third line   PHENOBARBITONE

              or

              CLONAZEPAM

(C)   **Absence**
     ('Petit mal')

First line   ETHOSUXIMIDE   0.5–2 g nocte
                                        0.25–1 g nocte (child)
              (sedation, GI upset, agitation and aggression; rarely
              blood dyscrasia)

              or

              SODIUM VALPROATE

              or

Second line CLONAZEPAM

(D)   **Myoclonic**

First line   SODIUM VALPROATE

              or

Second line CLONAZEPAM

3

Drug Treatment Policies

(E) **Febrile convulsions**

Immediate   TEPID SPONGING

and

ASPIRIN   100 mg/kg/day *divided* into
                                 4 hourly doses

or

PARACETAMOL   25 mg/kg/day *divided* into 4
                                 hourly doses

Prophylaxis SODIUM VALPROATE   10–30 mg/kg b.d.
(If frequent seizures or family history of idiopathic epilepsy)

or
PHENOBARBITONE   5–10 mg/kg/day

(F) **Status epilepticus**

First line   DIAZEPAM   10–20 mg i.v.
                                         0.3 mg/kg i.v. (child)
                                         5 mg rectally (infant)

or

CLONAZEPAM   1–2 mg i.v.
                                         0.5 mg i.v. (child)

or

Second line PHENYTOIN   10–15 mg/kg i.v. slowly
                (avoid if taking phenytoin orally)

or

PARALDEHYDE   5–10 ml i.m.
                                         0.5–5 ml i.m. (child)

GOUT

Administration of high doses of any effective non-steroidal anti-inflammatory will produce prompt resolution of pain and inflammation. Colchicine has been superseded because of gastro-intestinal intolerance. Long-term prophylaxis of hyperuricaemia should not be begun during or soon after an acute attack and should be accompanied by low dose anti-inflammatory drug therapy for the first 2 months of treatment to prevent recurrent acute gout. Patients taking prophylactic medication should also be advised to maintain a high fluid intake to prevent renal urate stones.

ACUTE ATTACK

INDOMETHACIN
50 mg q.i.d.

or

NAPROXEN 750 mg b.d.

until attack subsides and then tail off over 10 days

PROPHYLAXIS

First line ALLOPURINOL 200–600 mg daily

and

INDOMETHACIN 25 mg t.i.d. (for 2 months)

or

NAPROXEN 250–500 mg b.d. (for 2 months)

or

Second line PROBENECID 0.5–1 g b.d.

or

SULPHINPYRAZONE 100–200 mg b.d.–q.i.d.

and

INDOMETHACIN 25 mg t.i.d. (for 2 months)

or

NAPROXEN 250–500 mg b.d. (for 2 months)

HYPERTENSION

The management of hypertension has been revolutionised by the realisation that small doses of synergistic drugs will control blood pressure in most patients with few subjective side-effects. As blood pressure varies substantially repeated accurate readings should be made at separate visits prior to initiating therapy. Treatment should be initiated in patients under 70 years if diastolic pressure is greater than 100 mm Hg.

The end-point for the majority of treated patients is normotension, i.e. < 140/90 mm Hg but for those arteriopathic patients with very high systolic pressures (e.g. > 220 mm Hg) out of proportion to the diastolic pressure of 100–110 mm Hg, an attempt should be made to bring the systolic pressure to around 160 mm Hg. In patients between 70 and 80 years, treatment should be started only at pressures greater than 200/110 mm Hg or if hypersensitive complications such as cardiac failure are present. Patients over 80 years should *not* have antihypertensive treatment initiated.

Most patients with appreciable hypertension will require 'triple therapy' with a beta blocker, diuretic and vasodilator. Patients for whom beta blockade is contraindicated (asthma) or not tolerated (cardiac failure, claudication, cold extremities, fatigue, sexual difficulties) present a particular challenge. Some knowledge of the side-effects of the individual drugs and drug groups is essential in adjusting choice and dosage for the patient. Initial treatment is always restricted to a single drug to allow smooth titration of blood pressure reduction. Further drugs may be added over the course of the first few months of therapy

General measures

Weight loss
Salt reduction
Alcohol restriction

First line — Beta blocker

PROPRANOLOL 40–320 mg b.d.

or

ATENOLOL 50–200 mg daily
(COAD, cold extremities, insulin-dependent diabetes)

or

PINDOLOL 5 mg b.d.–t.i.d.
(bradycardia, previous cardiac failure, claudication)

Side-effects:

Cardiac failure, bronchospasm, bradycardia, fatigue, intermittent claudication, cold extremities, nightmares, impotence

and/or

Second line — Diuretic

BENDROFLUAZIDE 5 mg daily

or

THIAZIDE/K$^+$ SPARING DIURETIC COMBINATION
(DYAZIDE, MODURETIC, ALDACTIDE) if
hypokalaemia <3 mmol/l, symptomatic or normal
renal function on digoxin

Side-effects: Thiazides — hypokalaemia, gout, diabetes mellitus,
impotence, hyperlipidaemia, rashes, rarely blood
dyscrasias.
K$^+$ sparing diuretics — hyperkalaemia (all), impotence
and gynaecomastia (spironolactone), gastrointestinal
upset (spironolactone, amiloride) anaemia
(triamterene)

and

Third line — Vasodilator

HYDRALAZINE 25–100 mg b.d. (arteriolar
vasodilator)
or

PRAZOSIN 0.5–10 mg b.d. (alpha blocker)

or

NIFEDIPINE 10–30 mg t.i.d. (calcium antagonist)

Side-effects: Hydralazine — headache, tachycardia, flushing, lupus-
syndrome (rare).
Prazosin — start with 0.5 mg test dose as sudden
hypotension can occur with first dose; postural
hypotension, drowsiness headache, weakness,
nausea, vomiting, diarrhoea, palpitations, impotence.
Nifedipine — flushing, headache, palpitations,
weakness, peripheral oedema.

Fourth line — Alternatives

VERAPAMIL 80–240 mg b.d. (calcium antagonist)
(particularly useful if bronchospasm contraindicates
beta blocker)

or

METHYLDOPA 125–1000 mg b.d. (centrally acting
sympatholytic)

or

INDORAMIN 25–100 mg b.d. (alpha blocker)

or

Drug Treatment Policies

3

Fifth line   BETHANIDINE 10–20 mg t.i.d. (adrenergic neurone blocker)

or

CLONIDINE 0.1–0.4 mg b.d.–t.i.d. (centrally acting sympatholytic)

Side-effects: Verapamil — headache, palpitations, flushing, constipation, cardiac failure, cardiac conduction disturbances.
Avoid combining with beta blocker.
Doubles serum digoxin concentration.
Methyldopa — sedation, depression, dry mouth, postural hypotension, fever, diarrhoea, failure of ejaculation, rarely haemolysis, hepatitis, pancreatitis.
Indoramin — sedation, dizziness, depression, postural hypotension, failure of ejaculation.
Bethanidine — postural hypotension, bradycardia, diarrhoea, sexual dysfunction.
Clonidine — sedation, dry mouth, depression, fluid retention, bradycardia, cold extremities.
Dangerous rebound hypertension on sudden withdrawal.

Sixth line — Resistant hypertension

MINOXIDIL 2.5–25 mg b.d. (vasodilator)
(large dose of loop diuretic may be necessary to offset fluid retention. Usually used with beta blocker)

or

CAPTOPRIL 12.5 — 75 mg b.d. (angiotension — converting enzyme inhibitor)
(start at 6.25 mg daily dose to avoid first-dose hypotension)

Side-effect: Minoxidil — gastrointestinal disturbance, headache, flushing, palpitation, hirsutism, fluid retention.
Captopril — abdominal pain, loss of taste, rash, hypotension, hyperkalaemia, proteinuria, blood dyscrasias.

HYPOTHYROIDISM

Symptomatic hypothyroidism is common. Although it can present at any age, the major problems occur in the elderly with ischaemic heart disease. In such patients initial thyroxine dose must be low and timing of dosage increments carefully chosen. Optimal cardiovascular support with nitrates and beta blockers should also be prescribed.

Initiating treatment
THYROXINE 0.025 –0.05 mg daily initially.
Increase by 0.025–0.05 mg 2–4 weekly depending on cardiac status

with/without

ATENOLOL 50–200 mg daily, if angina (cardioselective, no hepatic metabolism, single daily dose)

Full replacement
THYROXINE 0.1–0.2 mg daily
Thyroid function tests including TSH should be normal after 3–6 months of thyroxine replacement.

IRRITABLE BOWEL SYNDROME

Diagnosis is made by exclusion following a normal full blood count, liver function tests, sigmoidoscopy and barium enema. Symptoms can range from simple diarrhoea through painful abdominal colic to intermittent constipation. Some patients require no active treatment following an adequate explanation of the nature of the disorder. Particular stress should be laid on the chronic relapsing symptoms and the fear of cancer allayed. Antidepressants should be restricted to patients with clear-cut depression. Long-term anxiolytics and neuroleptics should be avoided.

First line
Avoidance of obvious food precipitants
High roughage, high fluid diet

and/or

Bran 20 g/day

or

Fybogel 7 g/day

with/without

Second line   MEBEVERINE 135 mg t.i.d. before meals ⎫

or   ⎬ best used in short courses

COLPERMIN 1–2 t.i.d. before meals ⎭

or

Third line   LOMOTIL ⎫

or   ⎬ if painless diarrhoea

LOPERAMIDE ⎭

MIGRAINE

The underlying vascular changes in classical migraine with initial intracranial arteriolar constriction, platelet aggregation with serotonin release and later extracranial vasodilation provide the rationale for therapy with aspirin, ergotamine and, until recently, prophylaxis with the antiserotonin drug, methysergide. A particular problem occurs in severe migraine accompanied by nausea and vomiting due to gastric stasis. This impaired gastric emptying reduces substantially the rate of absorption of analgesics and ergot preparations, the latter of low bioavailability at best. The addition of oral metoclopramide, often combined with aspirin or paracetamol, to increase gastric emptying has been suggested but metoclopramide itself has to reach the upper jejunum to be absorbed. Amines in foods such as chocolate, cheese, citrus fruits and alcoholic beverages can precipitate headache. The oral contraceptive pill may provoke or exacerbate migraine and, in such women, there is an increased danger of cerebrovascular thrombosis. A progestogen-only preparation may be better tolerated by some patients.

Acute attack —Treatment is best begun at the onset of the aura

Drug Treatment Policies

(A)	MILD	SOLUBLE ASPIRIN	900 mg immediately 600 mg 4–6 hourly thereafter
		or	
		PARACETAMOL	1.5 g immediately 1 g 4–6 hourly thereafter
		or	
		MEFENAMIC ACID	750 mg immediately 500 mg t.i.d. thereafter
		with/without	
		METOCLOPRAMIDE	20 mg immediately 10 mg t.i.d. thereafter

(B) SEVERE   MEDIHALER ERGOTAMINE 360 μg (1 puff) immediately
Can be repeated every 5 minutes to a maximum of 6 inhalations daily and 15 per week

or

ERGOTAMINE TARTRATE 1–2 mg p.o. or p.r.
Can be repeated in 30 minutes
Maximum weekly dose should not exceed 12 mg
Once the headache has begun, ergot preparations are less likely to be effective and may even worsen the headache

and

METOCLOPRAMIDE   10 mg i.m. immediately
                                         10 mg t.i.d. p.o.
                                         thereafter

and

ANALGESICS as for mild attack

Prophylaxis   PIZOTIFEN   1.5–3 mg nocte
                                          or   0.5–1.5 mg t.i.d.
(side-effects include sedation, anticholinergic effects and weight gain)

or

PROPRANOLOL 20–80 mg b.d.

or

CLONIDINE 50–75 μg b.d.

or

DIPYRIDAMOLE 100 mg daily
(larger doses may provoke migraine)

PARKINSONISM

The central lesion in Parkinson's disease is degeneration of the dopaminergic pathways of the substantia nigra with subsequent depletion of dopamine. Treatment is aimed at restoring dopamine transmission. For most patients this is best achieved with the dopamine precursor levodopa together with a decarboxylase inhibitor which prevents the peripheral breakdown of dopamine and increases brain concentrations (Sinemet, Madopar). The smallest effective dose should be used and titrated upwards as necessary. Early in the disease, symptomatic improvement can be obtained with an anticholinergic drug such as benzhexol which reduces cholinergic overactivity secondary to dopamine deficiency or amantadine which inhibits dopamine re-uptake into the neurone. As the disease progresses, levodopa may become less effective and 'on–off' effects can occur. At this stage benefit may be obtained by the addition of bromocriptine, a direct dopaminergic agonist, or selegiline which inhibits the breakdown of dopamine. Bromocriptine can be used alone when levodopa is ineffective or poorly tolerated. Parkinsonism can be produced by treatment with antipsychotic drugs such as chlorpromazine and haloperidol which are dopaminergic antagonists. This may persist for weeks or months after the offending agent has been discontinued and is best treated with anticholinergic drugs.

First line   SINEMET PLUS   125 mg t.i.d. initially

or

MADOPAR   62.5–125 mg b.d. initially

Dosage should gradually be increased at weekly intervals titrating clinical response with the development of adverse effects. The final dose is usually a compromise between increased mobility and dose-limiting side-effects.

Side-effects: Anorexia, nausea, vomiting, insomnia, agitation, dizziness, postural hypotension, tachycardia, cardiac arrhythmias, involuntary movements, psychiatric upset

with/without

BENZHEXOL HYDROCHLORIDE 1 mg daily initially increasing to 2–5 mg b.d.–q.i.d.

Side-effects: Dry mouth, gastrointestinal upset, dizziness, blurred vision, confusion, tachycardia, psychiatric disturbances

and if deteriorating response or 'on–off' effect

BROMOCRIPTINE	1.25 mg nocte first week 2.5 nocte second week 2.5 mg b.d. third week increasing to 5–25 mg t.i.d. as necessary

Side-effects: As for levodopa, less nausea and vomiting but increased likelihood of involuntary movements and confusional states when combined with levodopa

and/or

SELEGILINE   5–10 mg daily

Side-effects: Nausea, vomiting, hypotension, confusion, agitation

and/or

DOMPERIDONE   10–20 mg t.i.d.–q.i.d.
(may improve levodopa absorption)

Second line   BROMOCRIPTINE

or

BENZHEXOL HYDROCHLORIDE

or

ORPHENADRINE HYDROCHLORIDE   50 mg daily
initially increasing to 50–100 mg t.i.d.

Side-effects: As for benzhexol but may be more euphoriant

or

AMANTADINE HYDROCHLORIDE   100 mg daily –
b.d.

Side-effects: Insomnia, dizziness, gastrointestinal disturbance, oedema, rarely leucopenia.

Symptomatic treatment of the dying patient involves the judicious use of appropriate drug therapy. The major problem is often pain and the fear of pain. Potent oral analgesics should be given regularly with the aim of keeping the patient pain free. An effective steady-state concentration should be maintained by ensuring that the dose is given before breakthough pain occurs. For many patients this is best managed by a flexible preparation such as morphine in chloroform water. Addiction is not a consideration and tolerance rarely a problem. Continuous treatment of other symptoms such as nausea, dyspnoea and constipation should be preferred to intermittent drug administration. Symptom control requires constant review as old symptoms may change and new ones develop.

Pain relief

Mild

SOLUBLE ASPIRIN	600–900 mg 4–6 hourly
or	
PARACETAMOL	1–1.5 g 4–6 hourly
or	
BUPRENORPHINE	200–400 μg 6–8 hourly sublingually

Severe

MORPHINE (5 mg, 10 mg or 100 mg) in chloroform water (10 ml)   5–10 mg 4 hourly
titrate as necessary up to 100–150 mg 4 hourly
(tolerance to drowsiness takes place over a few days)

or

MORPHINE SULPHATE CONTINUS (MST) 10–60 mg b.d.–t.i.d.

or

PHENAZOCINE   5–20 mg 4–6 hourly

with/without

OXYCODONE PECTINATE SUPPOSITORY 30 mg nocte

with/without

PROCHLORPERAZINE SYRUP 2.5–5 mg 4 hourly if nauseated
(can usually be disontinued after first week of morphine therapy)
If vomiting or unable to swallow:

DIAMORPHINE   5–30 mg 4 hourly i.m.

Drug Treatment Policies

3

ADDITIONAL PROBLEMS

Anorexia	PREDNISOLONE	15–30 mg daily
Bone pain	INDOMETHACIN	25–50 mg q.i.d.
	or	
	NAPROXEN	500–750 mg b.d.
	and/or	
	RADIOTHERAPY	
Confusion	HALOPERIDOL	5–10 mg i.m. then 2.5–5 mg b.d. orally
	or	
	THIORIDAZINE	25–50 mg t.i.d. (elderly)
Constipation	DORBANEX FORTE	5–10 ml b.d.
	or	
	NORMAX	1–2 capsules b.d.
	and/or	
	BISACODYL SUPPOSITORY	
	or	
	PHOSPHATE ENEMA	
	or	
	MANUAL EVACUATION	
Diarrhoea	LOPERAMIDE	4 mg stat, 2 mg after each loose stool up to 16 mg daily
	or	
	LOMOTIL	10 mg stat, 5 mg q.i.d. thereafter
Hiccough	CHLORPROMAZINE	25 mg i.m. or i.v.
	or	
	METOCLOPRAMIDE	10 mg i.m. or i.v.
Insomnia/ anxiety	DIAZEPAM	5–20 mg nocte
	or	
	HALOPERIDOL	1.5–5 mg nocte
	or	
	AMITRIPTYLINE	50–75 mg nocte

Drug Treatment Policies

3

Irritant cough	METHADONE LINCTUS	5 ml 4–6 hourly
Nausea and vomiting	PROCHLORPERAZINE or or	5 mg 4–8 hourly orally 12.5 mg 8 hourly i.m. or i.v. 25 mg 8 hourly rectally
	or	
	METOCLOPRAMIDE or	10–20 mg t.i.d. orally 10 mg 8 hourly i.m. or i.v.
	or	
	CYCLIZINE	50 mg t.i.d. orally, i.m. or i.v.

If due to cytotoxic drugs, NABILONE   1–2 mg b.d.
If due to hypercalcaemia, PREDNISOLONE   30 mg daily
If due to increased intracranial pressure, DEXAMETHASONE 8–12 mg daily

Nerve compression	PREDNISOLONE	15–30 mg daily
Raised intracranial pressure	DEXAMETHASONE	8–12 mg daily
Seizures	CARBAMAZEPINE	200 mg b.d. increasing as required to 600 mg t.i.d.

or

SODIUM VALPROATE 200 mg b.d.–t.i.d. increasing as required to 1 g b.d.–t.i.d.

and

DEXAMETHASONE (if cerebral metastases)

Terminal restlessness	DIAMORPHINE	10–20 mg	i.m.
	and		4–8 hourly
	METHOTRIMEPRAZINE	50 mg	

THYROTOXICOSIS

Medical treatment of thyrotoxicosis is largely confined to young patients with relatively small goitres. Surgery or radioactive iodine may be employed de novo if the goitre is large or the patient middle-aged or elderly. Antithyroid drugs have an 0.5% incidence of agranulocytosis. Routine WBC counts are not necessary but should be done if the patient presents with sore throat. Beta blockers with partial agonist activity (acebutolol, oxprenolol and pindolol) should be avoided. Concomitant thyroxine is also customarily prescribed to prevent glandular enlargement consequent upon increased pituitary release of TSH once the patient has been made euthyroid.

Induction of remission

First line	CARBIMAZOLE	40–60 mg once daily or divided doses for 1–3 months until biochemically euthyroid
	or	
Second line	PROPYLTHIOURACIL	300–450 mg once daily or divided doses for 1–3 months until biochemically euthyroid
	and	
Symptomatic	NADOLOL	80–240 mg daily symptomatically

(no intrinsic sympathomimetic activity, cardioselectivity or hepatic metabolism)

Maintenance therapy

Antithyroid drug dosage should be reduced slowly to a final small daily maintenance dose while retaining biochemical euthyroidism.

e.g. CARBIMAZOLE	5–15 mg daily	⎫
or		for 1–2 years
PROPYLTHIOURACIL	50–150 mg daily	⎬
with		
THYROXINE	0.1–0.2 mg daily	⎭

Attempt withdrawal

50% WILL RELAPSE ON ANTITHYROID DRUG WITHDRAWAL

then

FURTHER COURSE OF DRUGS

or

SURGERY (young patient, large goitre)

or

RADIOACTIVE IODINE (older patient, small goitre)

TRIGEMINAL NEURALGIA

First line CARBAMAZEPINE   100–200 mg b.d. initially
Increase dose at 2 weekly intervals till pain controlled. Initial side-effects of drowsiness, diplopia, headache, nausea and ataxia will occur unless dosage built up slowly. Final dosage may vary from 200 mg b.d. to 400 mg q.i.d. 33% fail to respond or cannot tolerate drug.

Second line PHENYTOIN   200 mg daily initially, slowly increased by 100 mg until plasma concentration > 10 mg/l, then by a further 50 mg every 2 weeks until pain controlled or toxicity occurs. Weekly phenytoin levels should be measured when dosage is being increased as metabolism is saturable. Reduce dose if ataxic or concentration > 25 mg/l

Third line CLONAZEPAM   0.5 mg b.d. increasing to 4 mg b.d.

Fourth line BACLOFEN   5 mg t.i.d. increasing to 25 mg t.i.d.

or

SURGICAL TREATMENT

ULCERATIVE COLITIS

Patients with ulcerative colitis who develop diarrhoea should be clinically assessed by sigmoidoscopy. Prompt effective treatment of mild attacks reduces the chance of progression to severe disease. Specific therapy should be provided and antidiarrhoeal agents should not be used. Steroids should be withdrawn if the patient is well and proctoscopy or sigmoidoscopy shows healing of the disease.

General measures

HIGH ROUGHAGE DIET
ORAL or INTRAMUSCULAR IRON (if necessary)

Mild attack

(Usually <8 bowel motions daily)

PREDSOL ENEMA
or
COLIFOAM

once or twice daily for 2–3 weeks

and

PREDNISOLONE

40 mg daily for 2 weeks then 20 mg daily for a further 2–4 weeks and slowly tailing off thereafter

and

SULPHASALAZINE

0.5–1 g q.i.d.

Severe attack

(Systemically ill, usually >8 bowel motions daily. As risk of acute dilatation or perforation, admit to hospital).

PREDNISOLONE

60–80 mg daily orally or i.v.

and

HYDROCORTISONE

100 mg b.d. as enema

and

SULPHASALAZINE

1 g q.i.d.

and

PARENTERAL NUTRITION
BLOOD TRANSFUSION
VITAMIN SUPPLEMENTS

as required

Proctitis alone HIGH ROUGHAGE DIET

and

PREDSOL ENEMA

or   b.d. until healed

COLIFOAM

and

SULPHASALAZINE   0.5–1 g q.i.d.

with/without

MEBEVERINE   135 mg q.i.d.

Maintenance therapy
SULPHASALAZINE   1 g b.d.–q.i.d.

Side-effects: Nausea, vomiting, abdominal pain, headache, vertigo, rash, reversible azospermia, rarely haemolysis, pancreatitis, Stevens-Johnson syndrome, photosensitisation.

Clinical Pharmacology Broadsheets

APPLICATIONS

This section tabulates the pharmacokinetic and pharmacodynamic features of the majority of important drugs in clinical use according to their therapeutic groups. For all drugs the half-life and disposition (metabolism and excretion) are included if the data are available. Specific information regarding mechanism of action (cardiac antiarrhythmics), indications (antibiotics), relative efficacy (analgesics), therapeutic ranges (anticonvulsants), dosage frequency (antihypertensives), side-effects (antipsychotic drugs) and pharmacodynamic properties (beta blockers) are quoted as appropriate. Relevant remarks regarding toxicity, active metabolites, inducing or inhibiting properties have been added. This aims to provide an 'instant replay' of the basic pharmacology of each drug allowing the prescriber to place it immediately in therapeutic and pharmacological context. This sort of data, coupled with the prescribing information found in the British National Formulary, will help in the choice of alternative medication for a patient intolerant to that initially prescribed, will facilitate appropriate dosage adjustment in patients with renal or hepatic impairment and will encourage recognition of potential adverse interactions between drugs following similar routes of elimination. The need for a higher dose may be anticipated when an enzyme inducer such as rifampicin or phenobarbitone is co-prescribed or a potential inhibitory interaction avoided in a patient receiving cimetidine or erythromycin. A knowledge and understanding of the clinical pharmacology of the drugs commonly employed can only improve and refine prescribing practice.

Analgesics

Drug	Half-Life (hours)	Disposition	Analgesic effect	Remarks
Aspirin (many)	0.3	Hydrolysed and conjugated Dose-dependent metabolism	+	Active metabolite — salicylic acid (half-life 3–6 hours)
Buprenorphine	3	Hepatic metabolism High first pass	+ +	Sublingual and parenteral preparations. Partial opioid agonist
Codeine	3–4	Hepatic metabolism	+ +	Morphine a minor metabolite Constipation likely
Dextromoramide	Not available	Hepatic metabolism	+ + +	Very short acting Used for 'breakthrough' pain
Dextroprop-oxyphene	12	Hepatic metabolism High first pass	+	Enzyme inhibitor Active metabolite Combined with paracetamol in Distalgesic
Diamorphine	Very rapid	Hydrolysed to morphine	+ + +	Particularly effective parenterally Activity due to morphine
Dihydrocodeine	Not available	Hepatic metabolism	+ +	Nausea, constipation and dizziness most frequent side-effects
Dipipanone	Not available	Hepatic metabolism	+ + +	Effect lasts for 4 hours Less sedative than morphine
Levorphanol	Not available	Largely conjugated	+ + +	Effect lasts for 6–8 hours
Meptazinol	2	Largely conjugated High first pass	+	Partial opioid agonist Still under evaluation
Methadone	15	Hepatic metabolism	+ + +	Slow onset of action Accumulation may occur
Morphine	3–4	Largely conjugated High first pass	+ + +	Long acting oral preparation available Analgesic of choice in terminal care
Nefopam	4	Hepatic metabolism	+	Unrelated to opiates Avoid combining with paracetamol
Paracetamol	2–3	Largely conjugated	+	Well tolerated Hepatotoxic in overdose
Pentazocine	2–3	Hepatic metabolism High first pass	+	Often CNS side-effects Weak analgesic

4

Clinical Pharmacology Broadsheets

Analgesics *(cont'd)*

Drug	Half-life (hours)	Disposition	Analgesic effect	Remarks
Pethidine	2–4	Hepatic metabolism High first pass	+ +	Short duration of action Dependence can occur
Phenazocine	Not available	Hepatic metabolism	+ + +	Effect lasts 6–8 hours Less sedative and constipating than morphine

4

ntianginal drugs (excluding beta blockers)

ug	Half-life (hours)	Disposition	Mechanism of action	Remarks
pyridamole	2–3	Largely conjugated	Coronary vasodilator Decreases platelet adhesiveness	More commonly used for anti-platelet effects
yceryl nitrate	3 min	Hydrolysed in liver High first pass	Venodilator	Sublingual, inhaled or topical preparations
sorbide itrate	1	Hepatic metabolism High first pass	Venodilator	Effective sublingually, orally or intravenously as infusion
sorbide nonitrate	5	Hepatic metabolism	Venodilator	Metabolite of isosorbide dinitrate. 100% bioavailability
edipine	4–5	Hepatic metabolism	Calcium antagonist	May increase heart rate
ntaerythritol anitrate	3–5	Hepatic metabolism High first pass	Venodilator	Marked variation in bioavailability
hexiline	2–6 days	Hepatic metabolism	Unknown; behaves like calcium antagonist	Prohibitive side-effects
nylamine	7	Hepatic metabolism	Depletes catecholamine stores; some slowing of calcium transport	Myocardial depression may be troublesome
apamil	3–7	Hepatic metabolism High first pass	Calcium antagonist	Also cardiac antiarrhythmic Avoid combination with beta blocker

4

Clinical Pharmacology Broadsheets

Antibacterial drugs

Type of drug	Drug	Half-life (hours)
Aminoglycoside	Amikacin Gentamicin Kanamycin Neomycin Netilmicin Streptomycin Tobramycin	2–3
Antituberculous	Ethambutol	2–4
Antituberculous	Isoniazid	1–3
Antituberculous	Pyrazinamide	10
Antituberculous	Rifampicin	1.5–5
Antituberculous	Streptomycin	2–3
Cephalosporin and cephamycin	*Cefaclor *Cefadroxil Cefotaxime Cefoxitin Cefsulodin Cefuroxime *Cephalexin Cephaloridine Cephalothin Cephamandole Cephazolin *Cephradine	0.5–1.5
	Latamoxef sodium	2–3
Macrolide	Erythromycin	1–3
Penicillinase sensitive penicillin	Benzyl-penicillin	0.5–1

4

Disposition	Bacteriological spectrum	Remarks
More than 90% excreted unchanged in the urine	Broad spectrum Severe gram negative infections	Not enterally absorbed. Reduce dose in conjunction with GFR. Ototoxicity and nephrotoxicity main side-effects. Plasma levels should be monitored. Neomycin used orally only in hepatic failure. Streptomycin a 2nd line antituberculous agent
Largely excreted unchanged	1st line	Reversible retrobulbar neuritis most important side-effect. Reduce dose if renal impairment
Hepatic metabolism Polymorphic acetylation	1st line	Enzyme inhibitor Minor liver function abnormalities in 20% patients. Occasionally severe hepatitis
Hepatic metabolism	2nd line	Hepatotoxicity a major problem
Hepatic metabolism	1st line	Potent enzyme inducer Implicated in hepatotoxicity when given with isoniazid
Excreted unchanged	2nd line	Ototoxicity and nephrotoxicity Monitor plasma levels
Largely excreted unchanged in the urine	Broad spectrum	Principle side-effects are hypersensitivity reactions Reduce dose if renal impairment Cephaloridine is nephrotoxic *oral preparations
Largely excreted unchanged	Broad spectrum	Can produce bleeding
Largely metabolised 30% unchanged in bile	Similar to penicillins Also mycoplasma	Enzyme inhibitor Estolate causes jaundice
90% excreted unchanged	Gram + ve cocci Actinomycosis Syphilis Tetanus	Hypersensitivity reactions include rashes, anaphylaxis, serum sickness, fever, arthralgia, angioneurotic oedema, and interstitial nephritis

Clinical Pharmacology Broadsheets

Antibacterial drugs *(cont'd)*

Type of drug	Drug	Half-life (hours)
Penicillinase sensitive penicillin	**Phenoxymethyl-penicillin**	0.5–1
Broad spectrum penicillin	**Ampicillin**	1–1.5
Ampicillin esters	**Bacampicillin** **Pivampicillin** **Talampicillin**	1–1.5
Broad spectrum penicillin	**Amoxycillin**	0.5–1
Penicillinase resistant penicillin	**Cloxacillin** **Flucloxacillin**	0.5–1
Antipseudomonal penicillins	**Azlocillin** **Carbenicillin** **Mezlocillin** **Piperacillin** **Ticarcillin**	0.5–1.5
Sulphonamide	**Sulphadimidine**	7
Sulphonamide	**Sulphamethizole**	1–2
Sulphonamide	**Co-trimoxazole** (sulphamethoxazole + trimethoprim)	8–12
Tetracycline	**Tetracycline**	6–10

Clinical Pharmacology Broadsheets

Disposition	Bacteriological spectrum	Remarks
90% excreted unchanged	Gram +ve cocci Actinomycosis Syphilis Tetanus	Hypersensitivity reactions include rashes, anaphylaxis, serum sickness, fever, arthralgia, angioneurotic oedema, and interstitial nephritis
70–80% excreted unchanged Some biliary excretion	Broad spectrum	Hypersensitivity reactions include rashes, anaphylaxis, serum sickness, fever, arthralgia, angioneurotic oedema, and interstitial nephritis
70% excreted as ampicillin in the urine	Broad spectrum	Pro-drugs Expensive ampicillin substitutes Lower incidence of diarrhoea
40–70% excreted unchanged in urine	Broad spectrum	Hypersensitivity reactions include rashes, anaphylaxis, serum sickness, fever, arthralgia, angioneurotic oedema, and interstitial nephritis
30–50% excreted unchanged in urine Significant hepatic metabolism	Penicillinase-producing staphylococci	Gastric acid stable Oral flucloxacillin preferred
70–90% excreted unchanged	Pseudomonas and proteus species	Not enterally absorbed Decrease i.v. dosage in renal failure Side effects as for benzylpenicillin
Hepatic acetylation 20–40% excreted unchanged	Severe urinary tract infections	Side-effects include nausea, vomiting, rashes, blood dyscrasias and hepatotoxicity
60% excreted unchanged in the urine	Severe urinary tract infections	Side-effects as for sulphadimidine
30–50% excreted unchanged	Severe urinary tract infections Chronic bronchitis Salmonella Brucella Pneumocystis carinii	Enzyme inhibitor Twice daily formulation Avoid in pregnancy Side-effects as for sulphadimidine
Largely excreted unchanged	Broad spectrum Chlamydia Rickettsia Brucella H. influenzae	Avoid in renal failure Deposited in growing bones and teeth

Type of drug	Drug	Half-life (hours)
Tetracycline	**Chlortetracycline**	2–6
Tetracycline	**Doxycycline**	14–20
Tetracycline	**Minocycline**	15–20
Tetracycline	**Oxytetracycline**	6–10
	Chloramphenicol	2–3
	Clindamycin	2–4
	Dapsone	10–50
	Lincomycin	5
	Metronidazole	6–14
	Nalidixic acid	1–2.5
	Nitrofurantoin	0.3–0.6
	Sodium fusidate	8–10
	Trimethoprim	10–16
	Vancomycin	6–11

4

Disposition	Bacteriological spectrum	Remarks
Largely eliminated by biliary excretion	Broad spectrum	Side-effects as for tetracycline
Largely metabolised 30% excreted unchanged	As for tetracycline	Can be given in renal failure Other side-effects as for tetracycline
Largely metabolised	As for tetracycline Also meningococcus	Side-effects as for tetracycline
Largely excreted unchanged in the urine	Broad spectrum Also acne vulgaris	Side-effects as for tetracycline
Hepatic metabolism	Typhoid Paratyphoid H. influenzae meningitis Klebsiella	Blood dyscrasias Enzyme inhibitor Avoid in pregnancy
Hepatic metabolism	Staphylococcal bone and joint infections Peritonitis	Major cause of pseudomembranous colitis
Hepatic metabolism Polymorphic acetylation	Leprosy Dermatitis herpetiformis	Contraindicated in pregnancy
Hepatic metabolism	As for clindamicin	Major cause of pseudomembranous colitis
Hepatic metabolism	Anaerobes Giardiasis Amoebiasis	Dose-dependent neurotoxicity Enzyme inhibitor
Largely metabolised	Gram negative urinary infections	Used for urinary tract infection only Mainly gastrointestinal side-effects
Mainly metabolised 30–40% excreted unchanged	Gram negative urinary infections	Side-effects include nausea, vomiting, rashes and rarely peripheral neuropathy, pulmonary infiltration and hepatotoxicity
Hepatic metabolism	Penicillinase-producing staphylococci	Particularly useful in osteomyelitis
40–70% excreted unchanged	Gram −ve species	Used for urinary tract infections and bronchitis
Excreted unchanged	Pseudomembranous colitis Resistant staphylococci	Nephrotoxic Ototoxic

Anticonvulsants

Drug	Indication (seizure type)	Half-life (hours)
Carbamazepine	Tonic-clonic Partial	25–45 (initial) 10–20 (chronic)
Chlormethiazole	Status epilepticus	3–5
Clobazam	Adjunctive treatment of partial epilepsy	18
Clonazepam	All generalised types	20–40
Diazepam	Status epilepticus	20–70
Ethosuximide	Absence	30–60
Phenobarbitone	Tonic-clonic Partial	48–144
Phenytoin	Tonic-clonic Partial	15–60
Primidone	Tonic-clonic Partial	3–12
Sodium valproate	Absence Myoclonic Tonic-clonic	10–16
Sulthiame	Partial	30

Disposition	Therapeutic range	Remarks
Hepatic metabolism	4–10 mg/l (17–42 μmol/l)	Active metabolite Enzyme inducer
Hepatic metabolism	Not appropriate	I.v. infusion in resistant status epilepticus
Hepatic metabolism	Not available	Benzodiazepine Active metabolite Less sedative than clonazepam
Hepatic metabolism	Not available	Benzodiazepine Active metabolite Sedative
Hepatic metabolism	Not appropriate	I.v. and rectal use in status epilepticus 3 active metabolites
Largely metabolised 20% excreted unchanged	40–100 mg/l (283–708 μmol/l)	Side-effects include headache, sedation, nausea, vomiting, aggression
Largely metabolised 25–50% excreted unchanged	10–40 mg/l (43–172 μmol/l)	Enzyme inducer Avoid as monotherapy
Hepatic metabolism	10–20 mg/l (40–80 μmol/l)	Enzyme inducer Saturable metabolism Impressive side-effects
Hepatic metabolism	5–12 mg/l (23–55 μmol/l)	Phenobarbitone is a major metabolite
Hepatic metabolism	50–100 mg/l (347–693 μmol/l)	Enzyme inhibitor Rarely hepatotoxicity, thrombocytopenia and pancreatitis
60–70% excreted unchanged in urine	Not available	Enzyme inhibitor Low efficacy and impressive side-effects

Antidepressants

Drug	Basic structure	Half-life (hours)	Disposition	Remarks
Amitriptyline	Tricyclic	17–40	Hepatic metabolism High first pass	Active metabolite-nortriptyline Sedative
Clomipramine	Tricyclic	17–28	Hepatic metabolism High first pass	Active metabolite Also used for cataplexy
Desipramine	Tricyclic	15–23	Hepatic metabolism	Major metabolite of imipramine
Dothiepin	Tricyclic	50	Hepatic metabolism High first pass	Active metabolite Sedative
Doxepin	Tricyclic	8–24	Hepatic metabolism	Active metabolite Sedative
Flupenthixol	Phenothiazine	15	Hepatic metabolism	Dopaminergic antagonist Use if psychotic element
Fluphenazine	Phenothiazine	24	Hepatic metabolism	Dopaminergic antagonist Use if psychotic element
Imipramine	Tricyclic	9–24	Hepatic metabolism High first pass	Active metabolite Enzyme inhibitor
Lithium	Lithium carbonate	13–33	Excreted unchanged in the urine	Renal and CNS toxicity Therapeutic range 4–11 mg/l (0.6–1.6 μmol/l) Used in mania and bipolar depression
Maprotiline	Tetracyclic	21	Hepatic metabolism	Epileptogenic Minimal anticholinergic activity
Mianserin	Tetracyclic	14–33	Hepatic metabolism	Sedative Minimal anticholinergic activity
Nomifensine	Tetra hydroiso-quinoline	3–5	Hepatic metabolism 20% excreted unchanged	Active metabolite Minimal anticholinergic activity Dopaminergic agonist properties useful in depressed Parkinsonian patient
Nortriptyline	Tricyclic	18–93	Hepatic metabolism	Stimulant Enzyme inhibitor
Phenelzine	Monoamine oxidase inhibitor	Not available	Hepatic metabolism Polymorphic acetylation	Avoid tyramine-containing foods Prolonged biological effect
Protriptyline	Tricyclic	55–124	Hepatic metabolism	Stimulant

Antidepressants (cont'd)

Drug	Basic structure	Half-life (hours)	Disposition	Remarks
Tranylcypromine	Monoamine oxidase inhibitor	Not available	Hepatic metabolism	Avoid tyramine-containing foods Prolonged biological effect
Trazodone	Triazolopyridine	8	Hepatic metabolism	Sedative Minimal anticholinic activity
Tryptophan	Amino acid	3	Hepatic metabolism	Doubtful efficacy
Viloxazine	Oxazine	2–5	Hepatic metabolism	Minimal anticholinergic activity

Antifungal, antimalarial and antiviral drugs

Drug	Mechanism of action	Half-life (hours)	Disposition	Remarks
Acyclovir	Antiviral	3	Mainly excreted unchanged in urine	Used for herpes simplex and zoster
Amantadine	Antiviral	15	Mainly excreted unchanged in urine	Treatment and prophylaxis of influenza A. Also in Parkinsonism
Amodiaquine	Antimalarial	50	Excreted unchanged	Side-effects nausea, vomiting and diarrhoea
Amphotericin	Antifungal	24	Hepatic metabolism	Nephrotoxic Poor oral absorption
Chloroquine	Antimalarial	48	Up to 70% excreted unchanged in urine	Side-effects include nausea, vomiting, diarrhoea, headache, rashes, pruritus, psychosis, seizures and corneal and retinal damage
Flucytosine	Antifungal	3–6	90% excreted unchanged	Synergistic with amphotericin
Griseofulvin	Antifungal	10–24	Hepatic metabolism	Poorly absorbed Enzyme inducer
Hydroxy-chloroquine	Antimalarial	72	Largely metabolised	Side-effects as for chloroquine
Ketoconazole	Antifungal	6–10	Largely metabolised	Enzyme inhibitor Avoid in pregnancy

4

Clinical Pharmacology Broadsheets

Antifungal, antimalarial and antiviral drugs *(cont'd)*

Drug	Basic structure	Half-life	Disposition	Remarks
Miconazole	Antifungal	20–24	Largely metabolised	Enzyme inhibitor Causes hyponatraemia
Nystatin	Antifungal	Not given systemically	Not orally absorbed	Topical use in skin, gastrointestinal tract and vagina
Proguanil	Antimalarial	Short	Hepatic metabolism 50% excreted unchanged	Given daily as prophylactic Active metabolite, cycloguanil
Primaquine	Antimalarial	4–6	Hepatic metabolism	Haemolysis in glucose-6-phosphate dehydrogenase deficiency
Pyrimethamine	Antimalarial	36–120	Hepatic metabolism	Given once weekly as prophylaxis
Quinine	Antimalarial	5–16	Hepatic metabolism	Toxic to eye and ear
Vidarabine	Antiviral	3–4	Largely metabolised	Intravenous administration for systemic herpes infection

Antihistamines

Drug	Formulations	Half-life (hours)	Disposition	Remarks
Astemizole	Tablets	19 days	Hepatic metabolism	Less sedative Little anticholinergic activity
Azatidine	Tablets Syrup	8–9	Hepatic conjugation	Sedative effects potentiated by ethanol
Brompheniramine	Tablets Elixir Slow release tablets	15 (30–32)	Hepatic metabolism	Sedative effects potentiated by ethanol
Chlorpheniramine	Tablets Syrup Slow release tablets Injection	12–15	Hepatic metabolism	Intermediate sedation Injection used for allergic emergencies
Clemastine	Tablets Elixir	Not available	Hepatic metabolism	Sedative effects potentiated by ethanol
Cyclizine	Tablets Injection	Short	Hepatic metabolism	Intermediate sedation Used as anti-emetic

Antihistamines *(cont'd)*

Drug	Formulations	Half-life (hours)	Disposition	Remarks
Cyproheptadine	Tablets Syrup	Not available	Mainly hepatic metabolism Some renal elimination	Also used as appetite stimulant May inhibit lactation
Dimethindene	Slow release tablets	Short	Hepatic metabolism	Sedative effects potentiated by ethanol
Diphenhydramine	Capsules	4–8	Hepatic metabolism Substantial first pass	Sedative effects potentiated by ethanol
Diphenylpyraline	Slow release capsules	24–40	Largely hepatic metabolism Some renal elimination	Sedative effects potentiated by by ethanol
Ketotifen	Capsules Tablets Elixir	3	Hepatic metabolism	Sedative Anticholinergic Used in prophylaxis of asthma
Mebhydrolin	Tablets Suspension	4	Hepatic metabolism	Sedative Rarely neutropenia
Mepyramine	Tablets	Short	Hepatic metabolism	Sedative effects potentiated by ethanol
Mequitaline	Tablets	38	Hepatic metabolism	Intermediate sedation
Oxatomide	Tablets	48	Hepatic metabolism	Drowsiness Less anticholinergic effects
Pheniramine	Slow release tablets	Long	Mainly hepatic metabolism 25% excreted unchanged in urine	Sedative effects potentiated by ethanol
Promethazine	Tablets Elixir Injection	7–10	Mainly hepatic metabolism Substantial first pass	Sedative Anticholinergic effects
Terfenadine	Tablets Suspension	6–12	Hepatic metabolism	Less sedative
Trimeprazine	Tablets Syrup	6–12	Hepatic metabolism	Sedative effects potentiated by ethanol
Triprolidine	Tablets Elixir Slow release tablets	5	Hepatic metabolism	Sedative effects potentiated by ethanol

Antihypertensives (excluding beta blockers and diuretics)

Drug	Mechanism of action	Half-life (hours)
Bethanidine	Postganglionic blocker	7–11
Captopril	Angiotensin converting enzyme inhibitor	1–3
Clonidine	Presynaptic alpha agonist	8–12
Debrisoquine	Postganglionic blocker	11–26
Hydralazine	Arteriolar vasodilator	2–8
Indoramin	Postsynaptic alpha blocker	2–3
Labetalol	Alpha and beta blocker	3–4
Methyldopa	Central action	8–12
Minoxidil	Vasodilator	2–4
Nifedipine	Calcium antagonist	2–6
Prazosin	Postsynaptic alpha blocker	3–4
Verapamil	Calcium antagonist	3–7

4

Doses per day	Disposition	Remarks
2	Largely excreted unchanged	Largely superseded
2	Largely hepatic metabolism 35% excreted unchanged	Limited to refractory hypertension Impressive side-effects
2	50% metabolised 50% excreted unchanged	Sedative Rebound on withdrawal
2	Hepatic metabolism Oxidative polymorphism	Largely superseded
2	Hepatic metabolism Polymorphic acetylation	Lupus syndrome can occur in slow acetylators
2	Hepatic metabolised High first pass	Sedative Active metabolites
2	Hepatic metabolism High first pass	Primarily a beta blocker
2	Largely metabolised, partly in gut wall	Side-effects limit use
2	Hepatic metabolism	Restricted to resistant hypertension Fluid retention and hirsutism major side-effects
2–3	Hepatic metabolism	Potent vasodilator Use combined with beta blocker
2–3	Hepatic metabolism High first pass	Tolerance occurs Rarely loss of consciousness after first dose
2–3	Hepatic metabolism High first pass	Negative inotropic and chronotropic effects Avoid combination with beta blocker

Beta adrenoceptor antagonists

Drug	Half-life (hours)	Doses per day	Disposition
Acebutolol	3	2	Hepatic metabolism
Atenolol	6–9	1	Excreted unchanged
Labetalol	3–4	2	Hepatic metabolism High first pass
Metoprolol	3–4	2	Hepatic metabolism High first pass
Nadolol	14–24	1	Excreted unchanged
Oxprenolol	2	2	Hepatic metabolism High first pass
Pindolol	3–4	2	Largely metabolised
Practolol	6–8	1	Excreted unchanged
Propranolol	3–6	2	Hepatic metabolism High first pass
Sotalol	5–13	1	Excreted unchanged
Timolol	3–5	2	Largely metabolised

*Cardioselective drugs are preferable in patients with chronic obstructive airways disease, intermittent claudication and insulin-dependent diabetes.
†Drugs with partial agonist activity may be helpful in patients with resting bradycardia, risk of heart failure and cold extremities.

*Cardio-selective	†Partial agonist activity	Remarks
+	+ +	Active metabolite diacetolol — renally excreted
+	0	Dosage range 50–200 mg daily
0	0	Alpha-blocking activity but beta:alpha = 3:1
+	0	Poor oxidisers have higher concentrations
0	0	Very long acting
0	+ +	Dosage range 80–240 mg twice daily
0	+ + +	Active metabolite
+ +	+ +	Intravenous use only
0	0	Active metabolite — 4-hydroxypropranolol
0	0	Particular anti-arrhythmic properties
Un-certain	0	Topical use in glaucoma

Drug	Mechanism of action	Half-life (hours)	Disposition	Remarks
Aminophylline	Phosphodiesterase inhibitor Adenosine antagonist	3–9	Hepatic metabolism	Theophylline active metabolite Therapeutic range 10–20 mg/l (56–111 μmol/l)
Beclomethasone dipropionate	Glucocorticoid	5–10	Hepatic metabolism	Used prophylactically inhaled Can be given twice daily
Betamethasone valerate	Glucocorticoid	5–10	Hepatic metabolism	Used prophylactically inhaled Can be given twice daily
Budesonide	Glucocorticoid	Not available	Hepatic metabolism High first pass	Used prophylactically inhaled Can be given twice daily
Cromoglycate	Mast cell stabiliser	1.5	Excreted unchanged	Used prophylactically inhaled in extrinsic and exercise-induced asthma
Fenoterol	β_2 agonist	7	Conjugated	Inhaled Local effect only
Ipratropium bromide	Anticholinergic	3–4	75% excreted unchanged 25% hepatic metabolism	Inhaled only Useful in chronic bronchitis
Ketotifen	Antihistamine	3	Hepatic metabolism	Used prophylactically Not yet established
Orciprenaline	Partially selective beta agonist	6	Conjugated	More likely to cause cardiac arrhythmias
Pirbuterol	β_2 agonist	4–6	Conjugated	Inhaled and oral preparations
Prednisolone	Glucocorticoid	2–3.5	Hepatic metabolism	Long biological half-life
Prednisone	Glucocorticoid	1	Hepatic metabolism	Prednisolone is active metabolite
Reproterol	β_2 agonist	Not available	Conjugated	Inhaled and oral preparations
Rimiterol	β_2 agonist	Not available	Conjugated	Inhaled Local effect only

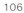

Bronchodilators *(cont'd)*

Drug	Mechanism of action	Half-life (hours)	Disposition	Remarks
Salbutamol	β_2 agonist	2–7	Conjugated	Tremor commonest side-effect Inhaled, oral and intravenous preparations
Terbutaline	β_2 agonist	3–4	Conjugated	Tremor commonest side-effect Inhaled, oral and intravenous preparations
Theophylline	Phosphodiesterase inhibitor Adenosine antagonist	3–9	Hepatic metabolism	Slow-release preparations preferred Therapeutic range 10–20 mg/l (56–111 μmol/l)

Clinical Pharmacology Broadsheets

Cardiac antiarrythmics

Drug	Mechanism of action	Half-life (hours)
Amiodarone	Prolongation of duration of action potential	15–30 days
Bretylium	Widens action potential duration	5–10
Digoxin	Blocks A-V conduction	24–48
Disopyramide	Membrane stabiliser	4–10
Flecainide	Membrane stabiliser	14–20
Lignocaine	Membrane stabiliser	1–3
Mexilitine	Membrane stabiliser	10
Phenytoin	Membrane stabiliser	24
Practolol	Beta blocker	6–8

4

Clinical Pharmacology Broadsheets

Disposition	Indications	Remarks
Hepatic metabolism	Refractory supraventricular and ventricular arrhythmias	Toxicity confines use to refractory arrhythmias
Excreted unchanged	Resistant ventricular arrhythmias	Hypotension can be troublesome. Injection formulation only
Excreted unchanged	Atrial fibrillation and flutter	Therapeutic range 0.8–2 ng/ml (1–2.6 nmol/l) Hypokalaemia potentiates action
50% metabolised 50% excreted unchanged	Mainly ventricular but also supraventricular arrhythmias	Therapeutic range 2.4–7 mg/l (7.1–20.6 μmol/l) Anticholinergic side-effects
Hepatic metabolism 30–50% excreted unchanged	Ventricular and supraventricular arrhythmias	Reduce dose if renal impairment
Hepatic metabolism High first pass	Ventricular arrhythmias, especially following myocardial infarction	Therapeutic range 1.5–5 mg/l (6.4–21.3 μmol/l) Only for i.v. use due to high first pass effect
Largely metabolised	Ventricular arrhythmias	Therapeutic range 0.75–2 mg/l (4.2–11.1 μmol/l) Impressive side-effects
Hepatic metabolism	Ventricular arrhythmias, especially digoxin-induced	Therapeutic range 10–20 mg/l (40–80 μmol/l) Hepatic enzyme inducer
Excreted unchanged	Acute management of supraventricular tachycardia	Cardioselective Parenteral use only

Clinical Pharmacology Broadsheets

Cardiac antiarrythmics *(cont'd)*

Drug	Mechanism of action	Half-life (hours)
Procainamide	Membrane stabiliser	2.5–5
Propranolol	Beta blocker	3–6
Quinidine	Membrane stabiliser	5–12
Sotalol	Prolongation of duration of action potential Beta blocker	5–13
Tocainide	Membrane stabiliser	10–14
Verapamil	Calcium antagonist	3–7

Clinical Pharmacology Broadsheets

4

Disposition	Indications	Remarks
20% acetylated 50% excreted unchanged	Resistant ventricular arrhythmias	Therapeutic range 4–10 mg/l (17–42.5 μmol/l) Active metabolite N-acetyl procainamide
Hepatic metabolism High first pass	Prophylaxis of supraventricular arrhythmias	Non-selective No partial agonist activity
Largely metabolised 10–50% excreted unchanged	Prophylaxis of supraventricular and ventricular arrhythmias	Therapeutic range 2–5.5 mg/l (6.2–16.9 μmol/l) Reduces renal digoxin clearance
Excreted unchanged	Prophylaxis of supraventricular arrhythmias	Non-selective No partial agonist activity
Largely metabolised 20% excreted unchanged	Ventricular arrhythmias, especially after myocardial infarction	Impressive side-effect profile
Hepatic metabolism High first pass	Supraventricular arrhythmias	Contraindicted in sick-sinus syndrome Avoid combination with beta blockers

4

Clinical Pharmacology Broadsheets

Drug	Mechanism of action	Half-life (hours)	Disposition	Remarks
Amiloride	Small natriuresis Conserves K^+ at distal tubule	6–10	Excreted unchanged	Hyperkalaemia may rarely occur
Bendrofluazide	Inhibits Na^+ reabsorption in distal tubule	3–4	30% hepatic metabolism Largely excreted unchanged	Long duration of action Less effective than loop diuretics
Bumetanide	Inhibits Na^+ reabsorption in ascending limb of loop of Henlé	1–3	Largely excreted unchanged	Loop diuretic
Captopril	Venous and arterial vasodilator	1–3	Largely hepatic metabolism 35% excreted unchanged	Used in severe heart failure Impressive side-effects
Chlorothiazide	Inhibits Na^+ reabsorption in distal tubule	1–2	Excreted unchanged	Long duration of action Less effective than loop diuretics
Digoxin	Blocks A-V conduction Positive inotropic effect	24–48	Excreted unchanged	Hypokalaemia potentiates action Limited value in sinus rhythm
Frusemide	Inhibits Na^+ reabsorption in ascending limb of loop of Henlé	0.3–1.6	80% excreted unchanged 20% hepatic metabolism	Loop diuretic
Hydralazine	Arteriolar vasodilator	2–8	Hepatic metabolism Polymorphic acetylation	Primarily reduces afterload Valuable in congestive cardiac failure
Indapamide	Similar to thiazides	10–20	Hepatic metabolism	Very long duration of action No advantage over thiazides
Isosorbide dinitrate	Mainly venodilator	1	Hepatic metabolism High first pass	Primarily reduces preload Valuable in chronic left ventricular failure
Mefruside	Similar to thiazides	Not available	Hepatic metabolism	Active metabolites No advantage over thiazides
Metolazone	Similar to thiazides	8	Largely excreted unchanged Some hepatic metabolism	No advantage over thiazides

Clinical Pharmacology Broadsheets

4

rug	Mechanism of action	Half-life (hours)	Disposition	Remarks
azosin	Venous and arterial vasodilator	3–4	Hepatic metabolism	Sudden loss of consciousness can occur following first dose Reduces preload and afterload
ironolactone	Competitive aldo-sterone antagonist	4–17	Hepatic metabolism to active drug — canrenone which is excreted largely unchanged	Hyperkalaemia if renal failure Long biological effect
amterene	Small natriuresis Conserves K^+ at distal tubule	1.5–2.5	Largely hepatic metabolism	Active metabolites
pamide	Similar to thiazides	5–8	Partly metabolised Partly excreted unchanged	No advantage over thiazides

orticosteroids

rug	Half-life (hours)	Disposal	Equivalent potency	Remarks
etamethasone	6	Mainly metabolised	33	Synthetic glucocorticoid
ortisone etate	0.5	Rapid hepatic meta-bolism to hydrocortisone	1	Natural glucocorticoid with mineralocorticoid activity
eoxycortone valate	Not available	Not orally absorbed	Not applicable	Mineralocorticoid superseded by fludrocortisone
examethasone	2.5	Mainly metabolised	33	Synthetic glucocorticoid
udrocortisone etate	0.5	Hydrolysed in liver	Not applicable	Mineralocorticoid with some glucocorticoid activity
ydrocortisone	1.5	Hepatic metabolism	1.2	Major natural glucocorticoid
ethylprednisolone	4	Hepatic metabolism	6.2	Synthetic glucocorticoid Used for transplantation rejection
ednisolone	3	70% hepatic metabolism 30% excreted unchanged	5	Synthetic glucocorticoid
ednisone	1	Rapid hepatic meta-bolism to prednisolone	5	Synthetic glucocorticoid pro-drug
iamcinolone	1.2	Hepatic metabolism	6.2	Synthetic glucocorticoid

4

Clinical Pharmacology Broadsheets

Cytotoxic agents

Drug	Mechanism of action	Half-life (hours)
Actinomycin D	Interferes with RNA and protein synthesis	36
Asparaginase	Impairs protein synthesis	8–30
Azathioprine	Cytotoxic immunosuppressant	3
Bleomycin	Interferes with RNA and protein synthesis	9
Busulphan	Alkylating agent — damages DNA	Very short
Chlorambucil	Alkylating agent — damages DNA	1.5
Cisplatin	Alkylating agent — damages DNA	24–72
Cyclophosphamide	Alkylating agent — damages DNA	5–6
Cytarabine	Interferes with pyrimidine synthesis	2.5
Doxorubicin	Interferes with RNA and protein synthesis	29
Etoposide	Inhibits DNA and RNA synthesis	3–15
Fluorouracil	Blocks pyrimidine synthesis	11 mins (20 metabolites)
Hydroxyurea	Inhibits ribonucleoside diphosphonate reductase	4
Melphalan	Alkylating agent — damages DNA	1.8
Mercaptopurine	Purine analogue	1.5
Methotrexate	Inhibits dihydrofolate reductase	27
Procarbazine	Inhibits DNA, RNA and protein synthesis	7 mins

Disposition	Remarks
Largely metabolised	Myelosuppressive
Extrahepatic metabolism	Toxic to liver, kidneys, pancreas and CNS
Hepatic metabolism	Metabolised to mercaptopurine Potentiated by allopurinol
Excreted unchanged	May cause pulmonary fibrosis
Largely metabolised	Used in chronic myeloid leukaemia
Largely metabolised	Used in chronic lymphocytic leukaemia
Excreted largely unchanged	Dose related nephrotoxicity
Hepatic metabolism Active metabolites	Pro-drug Activated in the liver
Largely metabolised	Myelosuppressive
Hepatic metabolism Active metabolites	Dose-dependent cardiotoxicity
Hepatic metabolism	Used in small-cell bronchial carcinoma
Largely metabolised Active metabolites	Used in solid tumours
Largely excreted unchanged	Myelosuppressive
Largely metabolised 10% excreted unchanged	Used in myelomatosis
Largely metabolised 20% excreted unchanged	Xanthine oxidase a metabolic pathway Potentiated by allopurinol
Excreted largely unchanged	Causes folate deficiency Folinic acid 'rescue' may be required
Largely metabolised	Antabuse reaction with alcohol

Clinical Pharmacology Broadsheets

Cytotoxic agents *(cont'd)*

Drug	Mechanism of action	Half-life (hours)
Thioguanine	Purine analogue	11
Thiotepa	Alkylating agent — damages DNA	Very short
Vinblastine	Arrests metaphase by disrupting micro-tubule assembly	2
Vincristine	Arrests metaphase by disrupting micro-tubule assembly	3
Vindesine	Arrests metaphase by disrupting micro-tubule assembly	24

Clinical Pharmacology Broadsheets

4

Disposition	Remarks
Largely metabolised	Induction agent in acute leukaemia
Largely metabolised	Used topically in malignant effusions
Hepatic metabolism	Causes selective leucopenia
Hepatic metabolism	Dose dependent neurotoxicity
Hepatic metabolism	Still to be fully evaluated

Gastrointestinal drugs

Drug	Mode of action	Half-life (hours)
Bismuth chelate	Local coating of ulcer	Not absorbed
Carbenoxolone	Increases gastric mucus production	15
Cholestyramine	Anion exchange resin	Not absorbed
Cimetidine	H_2 receptor antagonist	2
Codeine phosphate	Synthetic opiate	2–3
Diphenoxylate	Synthetic opiate	2–3
Domperidone	Dopamine antagonist	7
Loperamide	Local opiate and anticholinergic effects	7–14
Metoclopramide	Dopamine antagonist	3–6
Pirenzepine	Muscarinic antagonist	11
Ranitidine	H_2 receptor antagonist	2
Sucralfate	Local binding to ulcer base	Not absorbed
Sulphasalazine	Local antiinflammatory action	5–8

Clinical Pharmacology Broadsheets

Disposition	Remarks
Not absorbed	May blacken stools
Largely conjugated	Side-effects include hypokalaemia, fluid retention and hypertension
Not absorbed	Binds bile salts and also lipid soluble drugs and vitamins
50% metabolised 50% excreted unchanged	Enzyme inhibitor Reduce dose in elderly
Hepatic metabolism	Tolerance and dependence may occur with prolonged use
Hepatic metabolism	Combined with atropine in Lomotil
Hepatic metabolism High first pass	Less neuroleptic side-effects than metoclopramide
Hepatic metabolism	Lacks addictive potential
50% metabolised 50% excreted unchanged	Can cause dystonic extrapyramidal reactions
Excreted unchanged in urine	Occasionally dry mouth and visual disturbance
50% metabolised 50% excreted unchanged	Diarrhoea, headache, dizziness, rarely occur
Not absorbed	Major side-effect is constipation Can bind other drugs
Azo-reduction by gut bacteria	Split in gut to sulphapyridine (side-effects) and 5-aminosalicylic acid (local antiinflammatory action)

4

Clinical Pharmacology Broadsheets

Hypnotics and tranquillisers

Drug	Half-life (hours)	Disposition
Alprazolam	10–12	Hepatic metabolism
Bromazepam	8–19	Hepatic metabolism
Chloral hydrate	8	Hepatic metabolism
Chlordiazepoxide	6–28	Hepatic metabolism
Chlormethiazole	3–5	Hepatic metabolism
Clobazam	18	Hepatic metabolism
Clorazepate	Very rapid (metabolite 50–100)	Converted in stomach to desmethyldiazepam
Diazepam	20–70	Hepatic metabolism
Dichloralphenazone	Not available	Dissociates to form chloral hydrate and antipyrine
Flunitrazepam	20–36	Hepatic metabolism
Flurazepam	1–2 (metabolite 50–100)	Hepatic metabolism
Ketazolam	15–100	Hepatic metabolism
Loprazolam	4–8	Hepatic metabolism
Lorazepam	7–17	Largely conjugated
Lormetazepam	10	Hepatic metabolism
Medazepam	1–2	Hepatic metabolism
Meprobamate	6–11	Hepatic metabolism

Indications	Remarks
Anxiety	Benzodiazepine May have anti-depressant properties
Anxiety	Benzodiazepine Active metabolite
Insomnia	Active metabolites Gastric irritation may occur
Anxiety Alcohol withdrawal	Benzodiazepine 4 active metabolites
Insomnia Agitation (elderly) Alcoholic withdrawal	Dependence rarely Nasal irritation can occur soon after dose
Anxiety (elderly) Epilepsy	Benzodiazepine May be less sedative
Anxiety	Benzodiazepine Pro-drug
Insomnia Anxiety Alcohol withdrawal Status epilepticus	Benzodiazepine 3 active metabolites
Insomnia	Enzyme inducer Dependence can occur
Insomnia	Benzodiazepine Active metabolite
Insomnia	Benzodiazepine Active metabolite
Anxiety	Benzodiazepine Metabolised to diazepam
Insomnia	Benzodiazepine Active metabolite
Insomnia Anxiety	Benzodiazepine Intermediate action
Insomnia	Benzodiazepine Short acting
Insomnia Anxiety Alcohol withdrawal	Benzodiazepine 4 active metabolites including diazepam, oxazepam and temazepam
Anxiety	Minor enzyme inducer Dependence can occur

4

Clinical Pharmacology Broadsheets

Hypnotics and tranquillisers *(cont'd)*

Drug	*Half-life (hours)*	*Disposition*
Nitrazepam	30	Hepatic metabolism Polymorphic acetylation
Oxazepam	6–25	Largely conjugated
Prazepam	Metabolite 50–100	Metabolised to desmethyldiazepam
Temazepam	7–8	Hepatic metabolism
Triazolam	7–8	Hepatic metabolism
Triclofos	Not available	Hydrolysed to trichloroethanol

Clinical Pharmacology Broadsheets

4

Indications	Remarks
Insomnia	Benzodiazepine Prolonged effect
Anxiety Alcohol withdrawal	Benzodiazepine Intermediate action
Anxiety	Benzodiazepine Pro-drug
Insomnia	Benzodiazepine Short acting
Insomnia	Benzodiazepine Short acting
Insomnia	Similar to chloral hydrate

Clinical Pharmacology Broadsheets

4

Insulins

Type	Preparation	Manufacturer
Neutral (soluble but pH adjusted)	Actrapid MC	Novo
	Human actrapid	Novo
	Humulin S	Lilly
	Hypurin neutral	CP
	Neusulin	Wellcome
	Quicksol	Boots
	Velosulin	Nordisk-Wellcome
Biphasic	Initard	Nordisk-Wellcome
	Mixtard	Nordisk-Wellcome
	Rapitard MC	Novo
Zinc suspension (amorphous)	Semitard MC	Novo
	Semilente	Wellcome
Isophane	Isophane NPH	Boots, CP, Evans
	Human protaphane	Novo
	Humulin I	Lilly
	Hypurin isophane	CP
	Insulatard	Nordisk-Wellcome
	Monophane	Boots
	Neuphane	Wellcome
Zinc suspension (mixed)	Hypurin lente	CP
	Human monotard	Novo
	Humulin Zn	Lilly
	Lentard MC	Novo
	Monotard MC	Novo
	Neulente	Wellcome
	Tempulin	Boots
Protamine zinc	Hypurin protamine zinc	CP
	Protamine	Wellcome
Zinc suspension (crystalline)	Ultralente	Wellcome
	Ultratard MC	Novo

*emp = enzyme modification of porcine insulin
†crb = chain recombinant bacterial

Source	Onset of action (hours)	Peak activity (hours)	Duration of action (hours)
porcine	1	3–5	7
human (emp)*	$\frac{1}{2}$	3–5	7
human (crb)†	$\frac{1}{2}$	1–3	6
bovine	$\frac{1}{3}$	$2\frac{1}{2}$–$5\frac{1}{2}$	7
bovine	$\frac{1}{2}$	2–6	7
bovine	$\frac{1}{2}$	$2\frac{1}{2}$–$5\frac{1}{2}$	7
porcine	$\frac{1}{2}$	$1\frac{1}{2}$–$3\frac{1}{2}$	7
porcine	$\frac{1}{2}$	2–8	24
porcine	$\frac{1}{3}$	2–8	24
bovine 75% porcine 25%	2	4–12	21
porcine	$1\frac{1}{2}$	4–10	16
bovine	1	4–8	14
bovine	4	6–12	18
human (emp)*	2	5–11	24
human (crb)†	$1\frac{1}{2}$	3–8	19
bovine	2	6–12	23
porcine	$1\frac{1}{2}$	4–12	24
bovine	2	5–13	24
bovine	2	6–12	29
bovine	2	$7\frac{1}{2}$–12	29
porcine	3	7–15	22
human (crb)†	3	6–14	24
porcine	3	$6\frac{1}{2}$–$14\frac{1}{2}$	24
porcine	3	$6\frac{1}{2}$–$14\frac{1}{2}$	22
bovine	2	6–12	28
bovine	1	4–8	14
bovine	5	10–20	30
bovine	6	12–20	30
bovine	6	10–27	33
porcine	4	$9\frac{1}{2}$–$29\frac{1}{2}$	35

Neuroleptics

Drug	Chemical class	Half-life (hours)
Chlorpromazine	Phenothiazine	23–37
Clopenthixol	Thioxanthine	Not available
Droperidol	Butyrophenone	2
Flupenthixol	Thioxanthine	15
Fluphenazine	Phenothiazine	24
Haloperidol	Butyrophenone	13–40
Oxypertine	Phenylpiperazine	Not available
Pimozide	Butyrophenone	50
Prochlorperazine	Phenothiazine	4–5
Thioridazine	Phenothiazine	6–42
Trifluoperazine	Phenothiazine	2–12

Disposition	Side-Effects		
	Extra pyramidal	Anti-cholinergic	Sedative
Hepatic metabolism High first pass	+ +	+ +	+ + +
Hepatic metabolism	+ + +	+	+
Hepatic metabolism	+ + +	+	+
Hepatic metabolism	+ + +	+	+
Hepatic metabolism	+ + +	+	+
Hepatic metabolism	+ + +	+	+
Hepatic metabolism	+ + +	+	+
50% hepatic metabolism 50% excreted unchanged	+ + +	+	+
Hepatic metabolism Active metabolites	+ + +	+	+
Hepatic metabolism Active metabolites	+	+ + +	+ +
Hepatic metabolism	+ + + +	+	+

Neurological drugs (excluding anticonvulsants)

Drug	Indications	Half-life (hours)
Betahistine	Meniere's disease	Not available
Bromocriptine	Parkinsonism Acromegaly Hyperprolactinaemia Inhibition of lactation	3–5
Fenfluramine	Appetite suppressant	14–30
Levodopa	Parkinsonism	1
Mazindol	Appetite suppressant	12–24
Nabilone	Antiemetic	1–2
Orphenadrine	Parkinsonism	Not available
Selegeline	Parkinsonism	Long

Disposition	Remarks
Hepatic metabolism	Side-effects nausea, headache, and dyspepsia
Hepatic metabolism	Dopamine agonist Increase dose slowly to avoid toxicity
Hepatic metabolism	Risk of dependence Sedative and depressive
Tissue decarboxylation	Peripheral decarboxylation inhibited by benserazide (Madopar) or carbidopa (Sinemet)
Mainly metabolised	Similar adverse effects to dexamphetamine
Hepatic metabolism	Cannabis derivative Used during cancer chemotherapy
Hepatic metabolism	Anticholinergic side-effects
Hepatic metabolism	Selective monoamine oxidase inhibitor Safe with tyramine-containing foods

Clinical Pharmacology Broadsheets

4

Non-steroidal anti-inflammatory agents

Drug	Chemical class	Elimination half-life
Aspirin	Salicylate (salicylic acid)	0.3 (3–6)
Azapropazone	Pyrazolone	12–40
Benorylate	Salicylate	1–2
Diclofenac	Phenylacetate	1–2
Diflunisal	Salicylate	5–20
Fenbufen	Propionate	2–4
Fenclofenac	Phenylacetate	12
Fenoprofen	Propionate	2–3
Feprazone	Pyrazolone	24
Flufenamic acid	Fenamate	9
Flurbiprofen	Propionate	4
Ibuprofen	Propionate	2
Indomethacin	Indole	4–12
Ketoprofen	Propionate	2
Mefenamic acid	Fenamate	3–4
Naproxen	Propionate	12–15

Clinical Pharmacology Broadsheets

4

Disposition	Remarks
Hydrolysed and conjugated	Active metabolite salicylic acid Gastrointestinal intolerance major problem
Partly metabolised Partly excreted unchanged	Enzyme inhibitor Potentiation of warfarin, phenytoin, tolbutamide
Metabolised to salicylic acid and paracetamol	Biological half-life of its components
Largely metabolised	Longer biological half-life Given 2-3 times daily
Largely conjugated	Similar pharmacology to propionates Twice daily dosage
Hepatic metabolism	Active metabolites Given twice daily
Hepatic metabolism	Twice daily dosage Skin rashes a particular problem
Largely conjugated	Similar to ibuprofen 3-4 daily doses
Largely metabolised	Similar pharmacology to propionates but greater toxicity
Largely metabolised	Can cause diarrhoea
Largely metabolised	Similar to ibuprofen Headache and GI upset commonest side-effects
Largely metabolised	Available without prescription
Largely metabolised	Useful in gout Dyspepsia, headache, dizziness and confusion major side-effects
Largely conjugated	Similar to ibuprofen 2-4 daily doses
Largely metabolised	Promoted for dysmenorrhoea Can cause diarrhoea
Largely metabolised	Twice daily dosage Useful in gout

Clinical Pharmacology Broadsheets

Non-steroidal anti-inflammatory agents *(cont'd)*

Drug	Chemical class	Elimination half-life
Phenylbutazone	Pyrazolone	30–175
Piroxicam	Oxicam	35
Salsalate	Salicylate	3–6
Sulindac	Indole	7 (Sulphide 16)
Tiaprofenic acid	Propionate	2
Tolmetin	Indole	1–5

Clinical Pharmacology Broadsheets

Disposition	Remarks
Largely metabolised	Unacceptable risk of blood dyscrasia Restricted prescription
Largely metabolised	Once daily dosage Oedema may occur in elderly
Hydrolysed to 2 molecules of salicylic acid	Side-effects less frequent than with aspirin
Largely metabolised Sulphide active	Parent drug inactive Twice daily dosage
Partly metabolised Partly excreted unchanged	2–3 daily doses GI upset, headache, rashes major side-effects
Largely metabolised	Related to indomethacin but fewer side-effects

Oral hypoglycaemic agents

Drug	Mechanism of action	Half-life (hours)
Acetohexamide	Sulphonylurea Stimulates insulin release	1.3
Chlorpropamide	Sulphonylurea Stimulates insulin release	24–42
Glibenclamide	Sulphonylurea Stimulates insulin release	5–7
Glibornuride	Sulphonylurea Stimulates insulin release	5–12
Gliclazide	Sulphonylurea Stimulates insulin release	10–12
Glipizide	Sulphonylurea Stimulates insulin release	3–4
Gliquidone	Sulphonylurea Stimulates insulin release	1.5
Glymidine	Sulphonylurea Stimulates insulin release	2.5–5.5
Metformin	Biguanide Increases peripheral glucose utilisation	3
Tolazamide	Sulphonylurea Stimulates insulin release	7
Tolbutamide	Sulphonylurea Stimulates insulin release	6

Disposition	Remarks
Hepatic metabolism	Active metabolite Longer duration of action Once daily dosage
40% metabolised 60% excreted unchanged	Prolonged duration of action Avoid in the elderly Once daily dosage
Hepatic metabolism	Intermediate action 1–2 daily doses
Hepatic metabolism	Similar to chlorpropamide Once daily dosage
Hepatic metabolism	Single daily dose or taken with main meals
Hepatic metabolism	Single daily dose or taken with main meals
Hepatic metabolism	Very short duration of action Best taken with main meals
Hepatic metabolism	Active metabolite Once or twice daily dosage
33% metabolised 67% excreted unchanged	Rarely causes lactic acidosis Used with sulphonylurea
Hepatic metabolism	Active metabolites Once daily dosage
Hepatic metabolism	Short duration of action Largely superseded Metabolism inhibited by many drugs

5

Side-Effects of Drugs

INTRODUCTION

All drugs with pharmacological effects will have side-effects. These can be conveniently separated into predictable effects which are dose dependent and relate to the known pharmacological actions of the drug and idiosyncratic which are rare, bizarre, often fatal, reactions. Both types of adverse reaction can occur via pharmaceutical, pharmacokinetic and pharmacodynamic mechanisms. Examples of each of these are given below.

Mechanism	Predictable	Idiosyncratic
PHARMACEUTICAL	Drug delivery system may increase toxicity, e.g. small bowel perforation following osmotically-delivered indomethacin (Osmosin)	Excipients in the formulation may precipitate an allergic response, e.g. asthma induced by the yellow dye tartrazine
PHARMACOKINETIC	Individual differences in drug absorption, distribution, metabolism and excretion leading to high plasma levels, e.g. digoxin toxicity if renal function impaired	Toxic metabolite produced in susceptible patient, e.g. isoniazid hepatitis
PHARMACODYNAMIC	Altered drug sensitivity at receptor site, e.g. dystonia following low dose metoclopamide in children	Exaggerated tissue toxicity, e.g. chloramphenicol will cause reversible marrow depression in some patients but irreversible, often fatal, marrow aplasia in a few

Predictable adverse reactions are common and if recognised can usually be ameliorated by a reduction in dose or substitution by another drug. Idiosyncratic reactions occur in 1:1000–1:10 000 patients receiving the drug and may produce irreversible severe tissue damage, e.g. hepatotoxicity, nephrotoxicity, exfoliative dermatitis, peripheral neuropathy. Early discontinuation of the offending agent may abort the fully fledged toxic syndrome.

Recognition

The diagnosis of an adverse effect produced by a drug depends largely on recognition. This may be obvious when there is a clear-cut temporal relationship with the prescription of a new drug, e.g. an ampicillin rash. It may also depend on awareness of the side-effects of the prescribed agents, e.g. diarrhoea with mefenamic acid, negative inotropic effect of beta blockers leading to cardiac failure. Difficulties can arise when the adverse effect is similar to the disease treated, e.g. local skin sensitisation in a patient with otitis externa treated with neomycin-containing ear drops. Remoteness of the reaction in time from the original drug exposure may also be a confounding factor, e.g. hepatitis in an epileptic patient taking phenytoin chronically. Pathological deterioration in the function of a diseased organ may be assumed, e.g. cardiac failure precipitated by verapamil in a patient with ischaemic heart disease. Over-the-counter preparations must also be considered if a sudden change in the patient's clinical status is apparent or a new feature appears, e.g. hallucinations in a child taking a 'cough mixture' containing pseudoephedrine. The previous drug history may be helpful, e.g. aspirin-induced asthma. Combinations of drugs may potentiate one another's pharmacological effects, e.g. sedation with methyldopa and an antihistamine.

Suspicion of an adverse effect should be accompanied by a reduction in dose if it is an obvious pharmacological effect of the drug, e.g. sedation with amitriptyline. Pharmacological and chemical classes of drugs, e.g. phenothiazines, beta blockers, often share adverse as well as pharmacological properties. This can allow greater anticipation and earlier recognition of side-effects with a large range of similar drugs and is a major argument for generic prescribing. If an idiosyncratic reaction is considered, the drug should be discontinued immediately, e.g. penicillin rash. Rechallenge is rarely justified if alternative similar drugs are available.

Prediction

There are a number of factors which increase the potential for adverse drug effects. Although of great interest these are largely generalisations and are, as yet, unhelpful in predicting for individual patients.

GENDER — Females have a higher incidence of drug-related toxicity than males. This may be due in part to smaller body weight and in part to hormonal factors.

AGE — Drug handling and response may be impaired at the extremes of life. This is a particular problem in the elderly and is discussed in greater detail in Section 7.

HEREDITY — There are several genetic polymorphisms in drug metabolism which may increase the likelihood of adverse effects with particular agents. Acetylation and oxidation polymorphisms are considered in Section 1 under 'pharmacogenetics'. Histocompatibility status may predispose to adverse effects with gold and penicillamine and may be important in the development of drug-induced SLE. None of these factors are measured routinely and are currently of research rather than practical importance.

Side-Effects of Drugs

CLINICAL STATUS

Ill patients are more likely to suffer severe adverse drug reactions. Hepatic, renal or cardiac function may be intermittently impaired. They may be immunocompromised and often receive numerous drugs.

POLYPHARMACY

There is a substantial rise in the incidence of predictable adverse effects in patients receiving more than four drugs concurrently. Drug interactions are covered in Section 6.

ALLERGIC DIATHESIS

About 10% of the population are clinically atopic. These individuals manifest allergic drug responses more frequently than the rest of humanity. Particular problems are skin rashes and asthma.

Prevention

Probably the most important prophylactic measures involve careful prescribing and an appreciation of the pharmacological actions of the drugs used. Therapy should be started with small doses and response monitored wherever possible. Upward titration of the dose should be governed by response or the development of side-effects. Prescribing should be confined to a relatively few well-established agents. Particular care must be taken with drugs with a narrow therapeutic ratio such as warfarin, digoxin, phenytoin and for some of these therapeutic drug monitoring may be helpful in avoiding toxicity. The safest drug in any group should be employed, remembering that efficacy and toxicity are often directly related. Thus indomethacin may be an appropriate drug for a patient with rheumatoid arthritis but not for dysmenorrhoea. A knowledge of the expected problems with a drug is often invaluable in anticipating trouble. A patient pre-warned about the bronchoconstrictive effect of a beta blocker will not persevere when he begins to wheeze. Closer attention should be given to ill patients receiving a number of therapeutic agents and to the elderly. These precautions will help to reduce the incidence of predictable adverse effects. Idiosyncratic effects can only be avoided by abandoning the few drugs which are the biggest culprits, e.g. phenylbutazone, chloramphenicol. As most drugs can produce on a rare occasion a blood dyscrasia or a hepatotoxic reaction, such iatrogenic disasters will continue to occur. Early recognition with discontinuation of the offending agent may be life-saving.

Reporting

Serious adverse drug reactions with established preparations and all side-effects or possible side-effects with new drugs should be reported to the Committee of Safety of Medicines via the yellow card system. Problems with new drugs are of particular importance and these agents are indicated in the British National Formulary, MIMS and the Data Sheet Compendium by an inverted black triangle. Current estimates suggest that less than 1 in 6 serious adverse drug reactions are reported.

Using the tables

The following tables provide a convenient itemised list of the most common (predictable) and serious (often idiosyncratic) reactions to a number of well-established drugs. These are classified according to the system affected. Side-effects for each drug should be read across two pages. These tables cannot be fully comprehensive since many adverse effects are extremely rare and only become widely recognised after a prolonged period of drug use by a large number of patients. Similar chemical classes of drugs share many toxic effects and these can often be anticipated by a knowledge of their pharmacology. Thus, the corticosteroids, tricyclic antidepressants, phenothiazines, benzodiazepines, opiate analgesics, antihistamines and beta agonists are summarised in a single insertion. In addition, a selection of commonly used non-steroidal anti-inflammatory agents and hypoglycaemics are given as most of these drugs share similar side-effect profiles. Most recommended drugs and those figuring prominently in the drug treatment policies are included.

Side-Effects of Drugs

Analgesic and anti-inflammatory drugs

Drug	Alimentary	Cardiovascular	Endocrine	Eye/ENT	Haematological
Aspirin (also **Benorylate** **Diflunisal** **Salsalate**)	Nausea Dyspepsia Vomiting Mucosal erosion Peptic ulceration Haematemesis Melaena	Cardiovascular collapse	Ketosis Respiratory alkalosis Metabolic acidosis Hypoglycaemia	Tinnitus Deafness	Increased bleeding time Decreased platelet adhesiveness Hypoprothrom-binaemia
Corticosteroids	Peptic ulceration Haemorrhage Acute pancreatitis	Oedema Hypertension Cardiac failure Flushing	Sodium and fluid retention Hypokalaemia Hyperglycaemia Diabetes mellitus Adrenal suppression Growth retardation Amennorhoea	Corneal ulcers Raised intraocular pressure Reduced visual function Posterior subcapsular cataract	Increased blood coagulability Thromboembolic complications
Gold	Stomatitis Gastritis Colitis Peptic ulcer Glossitis Pharyngitis	Palpitations Flushing	Vaginitis	Keratitis Corneal ulceration	Eosinophilia Thrombocytopenia Leucopenia Agranulocy-tosis

Immunological	Nervous	Renal/Hepatic	Skin/Joint	Other	Drug
Angioneurotic oedema	Restlessness Dizziness Headache Mental confusion Coma	Renal papillary necrosis	Urticaria	Paroxysmal broncho- spasm Dyspnoea Sweating Hyperventila- tion Fever	**Aspirin** (also **Benorylate Diflunisal Salsalate**)
Increased liability to infection Masking of infection	Euphoria Depression Psychosis Intra-cranial hypertension		Osteoporosis Delayed tissue repair Subcutaneous atrophy Hirsutism Buffalo hump Increased bruising Striae Acne Hyperhydrosis Aseptic necrosis of bone	Increased appetite Moon face Muscular weakness Candidosis	**Corticosteroids**
Anaphylaxis Angioneurotic oedema	Peripheral neuritis Encephalitis Psychosis	Proteinuria Haematuria Nephrotic syndrome Hepatitis	Pruritus Rash Erythema multiforme Urticaria Eczema Seborrheic dermatitis Lichenoid eruptions Alopecia Exfoliative dermatitis Photosensitivity	Fever Weakness Dyspnoea Pulmonary fibrosis	**Gold**

Side-Effects of Drugs

Analgesic and anti-inflammatory drugs *(cont'd)*

Drug	Alimentary	Cardiovascular	Endocrine	Eye/ENT	Haematological
Ibuprofen (also **Diclofenac Fenbufen Fenoprofen Flurbiprofen Ketoprofen Naproxen Tolmetin**)	Dyspesia Peptic ulceration Melaena Haematemesis	Oedema Hypertension		Tinnitus Blurred vision Toxic amblyopia Vertigo	Agranulocytosis Thrombocytopenia
Indomethacin (also **Sulindac**)	Dyspepsia Stomatitis Peptic ulceration Melaena Haematemesis	Oedema Hypertension	Hyperglycaemia Hyperkalaemia Vaginal bleeding	Tinnitus Blurred vision Epistaxis	Leucopenia Thrombocytopenia Aplastic anaemia Haemolytic anaemia Agranulocytosis
Mefenamic acid (also **Flufenamic acid**)	Gastric discomfort Peptic ulceration GI bleeding Diarrhoea	Fluid retention	Vaginal bleeding		Haemolytic anaemia Agranulocytosis Pancytopenia Thrombocytopenia Bone marrow aplasia
Nefopam	Dry mouth Nausea Vomiting	Tachycardia		Blurred vision	

144

Side-Effects of Drugs

5

Immunological	Nervous	Renal/Hepatic	Skin/Joint	Other	Drug
Angioneurotic oedema Bronchospasm	Headache Dizziness Nervousness Depression Drowsiness Insomnia	Impairment of renal function Hepatotoxicity Interstitial nephritis	Rash Erythema multiforme		**Ibuprofen** (also **Diclofenac Fenbufen Fenoprofen Flurbiprofen Ketoprofen Naproxen Tolmetin**)
Hypersensitivity reactions including precipitation of asthma	Depression Drowsiness Mental confusion Lightheadedness Insomnia Psychiatric disturbances Syncope Convulsions Coma Peripheral neuropathy	Haematuria Renal failure Elevation of liver enzymes Hepatotoxicity	Rash Urticaria Pruritus Alopecia Purpura	Weight gain	**Indomethacin** (also **Sulindac**)
Hypersensitivity reactions including precipitation of asthma	Headache Drowsiness Dizziness Nervousness Convulsions	Renal impairment	Rash Purpura		**Mefenamic acid** (also **Flufenamic acid**)
	Drowsiness Insomnia Dizziness Lightheadedness Nervousness Headache Euphoria Convulsions		Sweating Rash	Respiratory depression	**Nefopam**

5

Side-Effects of Drugs

Analgesic and anti-inflammatory drugs *(cont'd)*

Drug	*Alimentary*	*Cardiovascular*	*Endocrine*	*Eye/ENT*	*Haematological*
Opiates (including **Buprenorphine Butorphanol Codeine** Dextropropoxyphene **Diamorphine Dipipanone Methadone Morphine Pentazocine Pethidine**)	Dry mouth Nausea Vomiting Constipation Biliary spasm	Bradycardia Palpitations Hypotension Circulatory failure	Reduced libido Gynaecomastia	Blurred vision Miosis	
Paracetamol	Nausea Vomiting Anorexia	Cardiac arrhythmias			Haemolytic anaemia Pancytopenia Thrombocytopen
Penicillamine	Oral ulceration Stomatitis Anorexia Nausea Vomiting Pancreatitis Impaired taste			Tinnitus	Lymphadenopath Leucopenia Thrombocytopen
Piroxicam	Gastric discomfort Peptic ulceration Gastro-intestinal bleeding Nausea Diarrhoea Constipation Flatulence Vomiting	Oedema Palpitations Hypertension Cardiac failure		Vertigo Tinnitus	Reduced platelet aggregation Prolonged bleeding time Thrombocytopen

Side-Effects of Drugs

5

Immunological	Nervous	Renal/Hepatic	Skin/joint	Other	Drug

Anaphylaxis	Sedation
	Confusion
	Vertigo
	Restlessness
	Mood changes
	Raised intra-
	  cranial
	  pressure
	Respiratory
	  depression
	Convulsions
	Coma
	Hallucinations
	Dependence
	Excitement
	Vivid dreams
	Tremor
		Urinary
		  retention
		Ureteric spasm
		Hepatic
		  impairment
		Nephrotic
		  syndrome
			Sweating
			Facial flushing
			Urticaria
			Pruritus
			Contact
			  dermatitis
			Pain at
			  injection site
				Hypothermia
				Pulmonary
				  oedema
					Opiates
					(including
					Buprenorphine
					Butorphanol
					Codeine
					Dextro-
					  propoxyphene
					Diamorphine
					Dipipanone
					Methadone
					Morphine
					Pentazocine
					Pethidine)

		Renal papillary
		  necrosis
		Hepatotoxicity
		  (high dose)
			Rash		**Paracetamol**

Angioneurotic
  oedema
LE
		Proteinuria
		Haematuria
		Immune
		  complex
		  glomerulo-
		  nephritis
		Nephrotic
		  syndrome
		Cholestatic
		  jaundice
			Pruritus
			Urticaria
			Arthralgia
			Pemphigoid
			  eruption
			Exfoliation
			Impaired wound
			  healing
			Alopecia
				Fever
				Myasthenia
					Penicillamine

Angioneurotic
  oedema
Asthma
	Dizziness
	Headache
	Sedation
	Fatigue
		Hepatotoxicity
		Renal
		  impairment
			Rash
			Photosensitivity
			Stevens-
			  Johnson
					Piroxicam

Drug	Alimentary	Cardiovascular	Endocrine	Eye/ENT	Haematological
Amino-glycosides	Nausea Vomiting Diarrhoea Malabsorption	Myocarditis		Otoxicity	Eosinophilia Blood dyscrasias Bleeding
Cephalosporins					Eosinophilia Blood dyscrasias Haemolytic anaemia
Chloram-phenicol	Nausea Vomiting Diarrhoea			Optic neuritis	Blood dyscrasias
Clindamycin	Diarrhoea Pseudo-membranous colitis				Blood dyscrasias
Erythromycin	Nausea Vomiting Abdominal pain Diarrhoea				Eosinophilia
Ethambutol	GI upset				Leucopenia
Isoniazid	Constipation			Optic neuritis	Blood dyscrasias
Metronidazole	Metallic taste Nausea Anorexia Abdominal pain Diarrhoea Vomiting				Neutropenia

Immunological	Nervous	Renal/Hepatic	Skin/Joint	Other	Drug
Lymphadeno- pathy	Headache Neuromuscular blockade Peripheral neuropathy	Nephrotoxicity	Rash	Fever	**Amino- glycosides**
Anaphylaxis Lymphadeno- pathy			Rash Urticaria	Fever Bronchospasm	**Cephalosporins**
Angioneurotic oedema			Rash	Candidosis Fever	**Chlorampheni- col**
Anaphylaxis	Neuromuscular blockade		Rash Stevens- Johnson		**Clindamycin**
		Cholestatic jaundice	Rash	Fever	**Erythromycin**
	Headache Dizziness Hallucinations Peripheral neuropathy		Rash Pruritus Arthralgia Acute gout	Fever	**Ethambutamol**
LE	Headache Dizziness Ataxia Sedation Euphoria Peripheral neuropathy Convulsions Psychosis	Hepatitis Urinary retention	Rash Arthralgia	Fever	**Isoniazid**
	Headache Vertigo Ataxia Confusion Seizures Peripheral neuropathy		Urticaria Flushing Pruritus		**Metronidazole**

Drug	Alimentary	Cardiovascular	Endocrine	Eye/ENT	Haematological
Nalidixic acid	Nausea Vomiting Abdominal pain			Visual disturbance	Blood dyscrasis Haemolysis
Nitrofurantoin	Nausea Vomiting Diarrhoea				Agranulocytosis Haemolytic anaemia
Penicillins	Nausea Vomiting Diarrhoea	Vasculitis			Eosinophilia Blood dyscrasias
Pyrazinamide	Anorexia Nausea Vomiting				Sideroblastic anaemia
Rifampicin	Nausea Vomiting Abdominal pain Diarrhoea		Menstrual irregularities		Eosinophilia Thrombocytopen Haemolysis
Sulphonamides	Anorexia Nausea Vomiting Abdominal pain	Cardiomyo- pathy	Hypothyroidism		Haemolysis Blood dyscrasias
Tetracyclines	Nausea Vomiting Dyspepsia Oesophageal ulcers Diarrhoea				Eosinophilia Thrombocytopeni
Trimethoprim	Nausea Vomiting				Megaloblastic anaemia Agranulocytosis Thrombocytopen

Side-Effects of Drugs

5

Immunological	Nervous	Renal/Hepatic	Skin/Joint	Other	Drug
	Headache Drowsiness Vertigo Convulsions	Cholestasis	Rash Photosensitivity	Fever Myalgia	**Nalidixic acid**

	Headache
	Vertigo
	Drowsiness
	Nystagmus
	Neuropathy
		Brown urine
		Cholestasis
		Active chronic
		  hepatitis
				Fever
				Myalgia
				Pneumonitis
				Interstitial
				  fibrosis
					Nitrofurantoin

erum sickness
naphylaxis
E
		Interstitial
		  nephritis
		Hepatitis
			Rash
			Erythema
			  nodosum
			Exfoliation
			Stevens-
			  Johnson
				Fever
				Candidosis
				Bronchospasm
					Penicillins

		Hepatitis Dysuria	Rash Urticaria Arthralgia Acute gout	Malaise	**Pyrazinamide**

	Fatigue
	Drowsiness
	Headache
	Ataxia
		Jaundice
		Hepatitis
		Acute renal
		  failure
			Rash
			Urticaria
				Fever
				Orange
				  secretions
				Weakness
					Rifampicin

erum sickness	Headache
	Peripheral
	  neuropathy
	Psychosis
		Crystalluria
		Hepatitis
		Nephrotoxicity
			Rash
			Erythema
			  nodosum
			Stevens-
			  Johnson
			Bechet's
			  syndrome
			Exfoliation
			Photosensitivity
			Pruritus
				Fever
				Malaise
					Sulphonamides

gioneurotic
oedema
naphylaxis
E
		Renal failure
		Hepatotoxicity
			Rash
			Exfoliation
			Photosensitivity
				Enamel
				  hypoplasia
				Dental
				  discoloration
				Candidosis
				Fever
					Tetracyclines

	Headache		Rash Pruritus		**Trimethoprim**

Cardiovascular drugs

Drug	Alimentary	Cardiovascular	Endocrine	Eye/ENT	Haematological
Amiloride					
Amiodarone	Nausea Vomiting Metallic taste Weight loss		Hypothyroidism Hyper- thyroidism	Corneal deposits	
Beta blockers e.g. **Atenolol** **Nadolol** **Propranolol**	Nausea Vomiting Diarrhoea Constipation	Bradycardia Raynaud's Cold extremities Cardiac failure Heart block			
Bethanidine	Diarrhoea	Postural hypotension Oedema Syncope	Failure of ejaculation Impotence	Nasal congestion	
Bumetanide	Pancreatitis		Hyperglycaemia	Tinnitus Deafness	
Captopril	Stomatitis Loss of taste Abdominal pain	Hypotension			Agranulocytosis Neutropenia
Clonidine	Dry mouth Pancreatitis Anorexia Nausea Constipation	Fluid retention Bradycardia Raynaud's Rebound on withdrawal	Gynaecomastia Failure of ejaculation Impotence		
Digoxin	Anorexia Nausea Vomiting Abdominal pain Diarrhoea	Arrhythmias Heart block	Gynaecomastia	Visual disturbances	Thrombocytopeni

Immunological	Nervous	Renal/Hepatic	Skin/Joint	Other	Drug
	Confusion		Rash	Hyperkalaemia	**Amiloride**
Angioneurotic oedema	Headache Insomnia Tremor Vivid dreams Vertigo Peripheral neuropathy	Hepatitis Cirrhosis	Photosensitivity	Pulmonary alveolitis	**Amiodarone**
	Vivid dreams Insomnia Depression		Rash Alopecia Erythema multiforme	Bronchospasm Fatigue Fever	**Beta blockers** e.g. **Atenolol Nadolol Propranolol**
	Depression				**Bethanidine**
			Rash	Hypokalaemia Hyponatraemia Myopathy	**Bumetanide**
		Proteinuria Renal damage	Rash	Hyperkalaemia	**Captopril**
Angioneurotic oedema	Sedation Depression Headache		Rash Pruritus		**Clonidine**
	Confusion Headache Drowsiness Depression			Malaise Fatigue	**Digoxin**

Side-Effects of Drugs

Drug	Alimentary	Cardiovascular	Endocrine	Eye/ENT	Haematological
Dipyridamole	Nausea Diarrhoea	Hypotension			
Disopyramide	Dry mouth Constipation Dyspepsia Nausea	Cardiac failure Hypotension Heart block	Hypoglycaemia	Blurred vision	Agranulocytosis
Flecainide	Nausea Vomiting			Visual disturbances	
Frusemide	Nausea Diarrhoea Pancreatitis	Hypotension		Blurred vision Tinnitus Deafness	Blood dyscrasias
Hydralazine	Anorexia Nausea Vomiting Diarrhoea	Flushing Palpitations Angina Postural hypotension Vasculitis Oedema		Nasal congestion	Blood dyscrasias
Indoramin	Dry mouth		Failure of ejaculation	Nasal congestion	
Labetalol	Nausea GI discomfort	Postural hypotension	Failure of ejaculation	Nasal congestion	
Methyldopa	Black tongue Dry mouth Nausea GI upset Diarrhoea Constipation Pancreatitis	Oedema Bradycardia Postural hypotension	Gynaecomastia Galactorrhoea Sexual disorders		Haemolysis Blood dyscrasias

Side-Effects of Drugs

Immunological	Nervous	Renal/Hepatic	Skin/Joint	Other	Drug
	Headache Dizziness		Rash		**Dipyridamole**
	Headache Dizziness Insomnia Depression Psychosis	Urinary retention Cholestasis	Rash Arthralgia	Hypokalaemia	**Disopyramide**
	Dizziness				**Flecainide**
	Dizziness Headache	Hepatotoxicity	Rash Photosensitivity Acute gout	Hypokalaemia Hyponatraemia	**Frusemide**
LE	Headache Vertigo Peripheral neuropathy Depression Tremor	Hepatitis Urinary retention	Rash Urticaria Pruritus	Fever	**Hydralazine**
	Sedation Dizziness Depression		Rash	Weight gain	**Indoramin**
	Scalp tingling Paraesthesiae Headache Insomnia Vivid dreams Depression		Rash	Fatigue Weakness Cramps Bronchospasm	**Labetalol**
LE	Drowsiness Nightmares Depression Headache Paraesthesiae Parkinsonism	Hepatotoxicity	Rash Arthralgia	Fever Myalgia	**Methyldopa**

Side-Effects of Drugs

5

Drug	Alimentary	Cardiovascular	Endocrine	Eye/ENT	Haematological
Mexiletine	Nausea Vomiting Dyspepsia Hiccoughs	Hypotension Bradycardia Atrial fibrillation		Diplopia Blurred vision	
Minoxidil	Nausea	Oedema Tachycardia	Gynaecomastia Menorrhagia Weight gain	Conjunctivitis	Thrombocytopenia
Nifedipine	Nausea Vomiting Dyspepsia	Headache Flushing Palpitations Hypotension Angina (on initiation) Peripheral oedema Cardiac failure			
Nitrates e.g. **Glyceryl trinitrate Isosorbide dinitrate Isosorbide mononitrate**	Vomiting	Flushing Tachycardia Hypotension Syncope			Methaemo- globinaemia
Perhexiline	Nausea Vomiting GI discomfort	Flushing Syncope	Hypoglycaemia Weight loss	Diplopia	
Prazosin	Dry mouth Nausea Diarrhoea Constipation Vomiting	Syncope (1st dose) Postural hypotension Palpitations Angina	Impotence	Nasal congestion Blurred vision Tinnitus	

5

Side-Effects of Drugs

Immunological	Nervous	Renal/Hepatic	Skin/Joint	Other	Drug
	Drowsiness Confusion Dizziness Nystagmus Dysarthria Ataxia Tremor Convulsions				**Mexiletine**
SLE			Hirsutism Pruritus		**Minoxidil**
	Dizziness Paraesthesiae Depression	Hepatotoxicity	Sweating	Fatigue	**Nifedipine**

	Headache
	Dizziness
					Nitrates
					e.g.
					Glyceryl
					  trinitrate
					Isosorbide
					  dinitrate
					Isosorbide
					  mononitrate

	Headache Dizziness Ataxia Tremor Paraesthesiae Convulsions Parkinsonism Peripheral neuropathy	Hepatotoxicity	Rash Urticaria	Weakness Reduced libido	**Perhexiline**
	Drowsiness Depression Headache Vivid dreams	Urinary frequency	Rash Pruritus	Lethargy Dyspnoea	**Prazosin**

Side-Effects of Drugs

5

Cardiovascular drugs *(cont'd)*

Drug	Alimentary	Cardiovascular	Endocrine	Eye/ENT	Haematological
Procainamide	Anorexia Nausea Vomiting Diarrhoea	Hypotension Flushing			Agranulocytosis
Quinidine	Nausea Vomiting Diarrhoea Abdominal pain	Hypotension Heart block Ventricular arrhythmias		Tinnitus Visual disturbance	Thrombocytopenia
Spironolactone	Abdominal cramp Diarrhoea		Gynaecomastia Hirsutism Menstrual irregularity Impotence		
Thiazide diuretics e.g. **Bendrofluazide**	Anorexia Abdominal pain Nausea Vomiting Diarrhoea Constipation	Postural hypotension	Parotitis Pancreatitis Loss of libido Impotence Hyperglycaemia		Blood dyscrasias
Tocainide	Nausea Vomiting	Hot flushes Bradycardia Hypotension		Tinnitus Blurred vision	
Triamterene	Nausea Vomiting Diarrhoea Dry mouth	Hypotension			Megaloblastic anaemia Thrombocytopenia
Verapamil	Nausea Constipation	Flushing Bradycardia Heart block Hypotension Cardiac failure Peripheral oedema			
Warfarin	Nausea Vomiting Diarrhoea		Priapism		Haemorrhage

Side-Effects of Drugs

5

Immunological	Nervous	Renal/Hepatic	Skin/Joint	Other	Drug
SLE	Dizziness Depression Hallucinations Psychosis		Rash Pruritus Urticaria	Myalgia Weakness	**Procainamide**
Anaphylaxis	Headache Confusion Vertigo		Urticaria	Fever Dyspnoea	**Quinidine**
	Headache Drowsiness Confusion Ataxia		Rash	Hyponatraemia Hyperkalaemia	**Spironolactone**
	Dizziness Headache Paraesthesiae	Hepatitis	Rash Photosensitivity Acute gout	Hypokalaemia Hyponatraemia Thirst Muscle spasm Weakness Pneumonitis	**Thiazide diuretics e.g. Bendroflu- azide**

SLE	Tremor
	Dizziness
	Ataxia
	Impaired
	  memory
	Poor
	  concentration
	Paraesthesiae
	Convulsions
			Rash	Muscle spasm
				Interstitial
				  pneumonitis
					Tocainide

	Headache		Rash Acute gout Photosenti- tivity	Hyperkalaemia	**Triamterene**
	Headache Dizziness	Hepatotoxicity	Rash Arthralgia		**Verapamil**
			Rash Alopecia	Fever Teratogenicity	**Warfarin**

5

Side-Effects of Drugs

Cytotoxics and immunosuppressives

Drug	Alimentary	Cardiovascular	Endocrine	Eye/ENT	Haematological
Azathioprine	Pancreatitis	Hypotension			Leucopenia Thrombocytopenia
Bleomycin		Cardiorespiratory collapse (in some patients with lymphoma) Raynaud's		Stomatitis Ototoxicity at high dose	
Busulphan			Adrenal suppression	Cataract formation	Thrombocytopenia Haemorrhage Irreversible bone marrow depression
Carmustine				Optic neuritis	Bone marrow depression Thrombocytopenia Leucopenia
Chlorambucil			Adrenal suppression Azospermia		Reversible lymphocytopenia Irreversible bone marrow depression Neutropenia
Cisplatin	Severe nausea Vomiting	Tachycardia Hypotension	Hypomagnesaemia Hypocalcaemic tetany	Ototoxicity Ophthalmic toxicity	Bone marrow depression Haemolysis
Cyclophosphamide	Vomiting Haemorrhagic pancreatitis	Myopericarditis Cardiomyopathy Hypotension	Diabetes mellitus Thyrotoxicosis Myxoedema Azospermia	Blurred vision	Leucopenia Thrombocytopenia

Immunological	Nervous	Renal/Hepatic	Skin/Joint	Other	Drug
Drug fever Hypogamma- globulinaemia Reduced immune response	Meningitis Paraesthesiae	Cholestatic jaundice	Necrosis at injection site Polyarthritis Arthralgia	Respiratory depression	**Azathioprine**
Drug fever Anaphylaxis			Rash Pruritus Hyperkeratosis Nail changes Striae	Pneumonitis Pulmonary fibrosis	**Bleomycin**
			Contact irritant Cutaneous pigmentation	Interstitial pulmonary fibrosis	**Busulphan**
	Confusion Lethargy	Renal toxicity Hepatotoxicity	Necrosis at injection site Transient hyperpig- mentation	Pulmonary fibrosis	**Carmustine**
	Neurotoxicity Seizures Sensorimotor neuropathy	Cystitis	Contact irritant Cutaneous pigmentation	Pulmonary fibrosis Interstitial pneumonitis	**Chlorambucil**
Allergy Anaphylaxis	Peripheral neuropathy Seizures	Renal tubular necrosis Hepatotoxicity	Angioneurotic oedema	Wheezing Pyrexia Rigors	**Cisplatin**
Anaphylaxis Hypogamma- globulinaemia Reduced immune response	Depression	Haemorrhagic cystitis Renal tubular necrosis	Alopecia Urticaria	Interstitial pulmonary fibrosis Pneumonitis	**Cyclophos- phamide**

Cytotoxics and immunosuppressives *(cont'd)*

Drug	Alimentary	Cardiovascular	Endocrine	Eye/ENT	Haematological
Cyclosporin	Gastrointest- discomfort Nausea Vomiting			Gum hypertrophy	
Cytarabine	Nausea Vomiting			Corneal ulceration with ophthalmic application	Granulo- cytopenia Megaloblastic changes
Doxorubicin	Oesophagitis	Arrhythmias Cardio- myopathy Congestive cardiac failure		Stomatitis	Bone marrow depression Leucopenia
Flurouracil	Severe diarrhoea Gastric ulceration	Tachycardia Angina		Stomatitis Lachrymation Oculomoter palsy Nasal discharge	Leucopenia Thrombocytopenia
Melphalan		Oedema following regional perfusion			Neutropenia Thrombocytopenia
Methotrexate	Enteropathy Severe diarrhoea Anorexia Haemorrhagic enteritis Intestinal perforation			Mouth ulceration Stomatitis	Leucopenia Thrombocytopenia Bone marrow depression Megaloblastic anaemia

5

Side-Effects of Drugs

Immunological	Nervous	Renal/Hepatic	Skin/Joint	Other	Drug
Predisposition to development of lymphomas Allergy	Mild tremor	Nephrotoxicity Hepatotoxicity	Hirsutism Angioneurotic oedema Rash		**Cyclosporin**
Allergy Drug fever Anaphylaxis	Central neurotoxicity Peripheral neuropathy Paraesthesiae	Renal dysfunction Abnormal liver function tests Possible veno-occlusive disease of the liver	Myalgia		**Cytarabine**
Anaphylaxis Angioneurotic oedema		Red coloured urine Acute tubular necrosis	Alopecia Necrosis at injection site Thrombo-phlebitis Urticaria and other rashes		**Doxorubicin**
Anaphylaxis	Mental confusion Ataxia		Local inflammation and photosensitivity Pellagra	Apnoea Pulmonary oedema	**Fluorouracil**
Anaphylaxis	Local neurotoxicity with regional perfusion		Vesiculation of skin with regional perfusion	Interstitial pneumonitis Lung fibrosis	**Melphalan**
Hypogamma-globulinaemia Reduced immune response	Arachnoiditis Convulsions Intellectual impairment Coma	Portal fibrosis Cirrhosis Uraemia Acute tubular necrosis	Contact irritant Osteoporosis Photosensitivity	Teratogenicity Pneumonitis	**Methotrexate**

Drug	Alimentary	Cardiovascular	Endocrine	Eye/ENT	Haematological
Mitomycin C					Aplastic anaemia Leucopenia Thrombocytopenia
Mustine	Severe nausea Vomiting			Tinnitus Vertigo Deafness	Bone marrow depression Anaemia Lymphocytopenia Granulocyto- penia Thrombocytopenia Haemorrhage
Tamoxifen	Gastric discomfort	Oedema Deep vein thrombosis Thrombo- embolism	Hypercalcaemia	Retinopathy	
Thiotepa					Bone marrow damage Aplastic anaemia Thrombocytopenia
Treosulfan					Transient bone marrow depression
Vinblastine **Vincristine** **Vindesine**	Constipation Abdominal pain Adynamic ileus	Hypertension Raynaud's Myocardial infarction	Inappropriate anti-diuretic hormone secretion	Optic nerve damage Parotid gland pain	Bone marrow depression Thrombocytosis

Immunological	Nervous	Renal/Hepatic	Skin/Joint	Other	Drug
		Haemolytic-uraemic state	Necrosis at injection site	Interstitial pneumonitis Pulmonary fibrosis	**Mitomycin C**
Allergy Anaphylaxis	Peripheral neuropathy		Necrosis at injection site Maculopapular rashes Urticaria Thrombophle-bitis Erythema multiforme		**Mustine**
	Dizziness Headache Depression Confusion		Hot flushes Rashes Leg cramps Alopecia Dry skin	Vaginal bleeding Pruritus vulvae Tumour pain Fatigue	**Tamoxifen**
		Ureteral Obstruction Renal failure	Contact irritant		**Thiotepa**
			Alopecia Pigmentation		**Treosulfan**
	Seizures Malaise Headache Depression Psychosis Paraesthesiae Neuromyopathy Peripheral neuritis Sensorimotor neuropathy	Uric acid nephropathy	Alopecia Dermatitis Necrosis at Injection site Photo-sensitivity		**Vinblastine Vincristine Vindestine**

Endocrine drugs

Drug	Alimentary	Cardiovascular	Endocrine	Eye/ENT	Haematological
Bromocriptine	Dry mouth Metallic taste Nausea Vomiting Constipation Diarrhoea Haemorrhage	Postural hypotension Bradycardia Arrhythmias Palpitations Peripheral vasospasm Peripheral oedema Exacerbation of angina		Nasal congestion Burning eyes Diplopia	
Carbimazole (also **Propylthio-uracil**)	Nausea Gastric discomfort			Sore throat	Agranulocytosis Thrombocytopenia Aplastic anaemia
Chlorpropamide (also **Glibenclamide** and other sulphonylur-eas)	Nausea Vomiting Epigastric pain		Inappropriate anti-diuretic hormone secretion (chlorpropa- mide only)		Eosinophilia Leucopenia Thrombocytopenia Aplastic anaemia Agranulocytosis Haemolytic anaemia Pancytopenia
Clomiphene	Gastro- intestinal discomfort Nausea Vomiting		Reversible ovarian enlargement Cyst formation Heavier menses Spotting Hydatidiform mole	Blurred vision	
Danazol	Gastro- intestinal discomfort	Oedema	Amennorrhoea Changes in breast size Changes in libido Weight gain Clitoral hypertrophy	Deepening of voice	

Immunological	Nervous	Renal/Hepatic	Skin/Joint	Other	Drug
	Headache Sedation Hallucinations Dizziness Syncope Mania Depression Psychosis Dyskinesia	Raised liver enzymes	Rash Alopecia	Leg cramps	**Bromocriptine**
Allergy Drug fever	Headache Psychosis	Hepatitis	Rashes Arthralgia Alopecia		**Carbimazole** (also **Propylthio- uracil**)
Allergy	Dizziness	Hepatotoxicity	Parasthesiae Rashes Facial flushing (chlorpropam- ide only) Exfoliative dermatitis Eczema Photodermatitis Erythema nodosum Purpura Stevens- Johnson	Weakness	**Chlorpropamide** (also **Glibenclamide** and other sulphonylur- eas)
	Depression Insomnia Headache	Abnormal liver function tests	Hot flushes Urticaria Alopecia	Fatigue Mutiple births	**Clomiphene**
	Headache Dizziness Tremor Depression Sleep disorder	Changes in liver function tests Cholestatic jaundice	Hot flushes Sweating Acne Oily skin Hirsutism Rashes Muscle spasm	Vaginitis	**Danazol**

5

Side-Effects of Drugs

Endocrine drugs *(cont'd)*

Drug	Alimentary	Cardiovascular	Endocrine	Eye/ENT	Haematological
Metformin	Metallic taste Anorexia Nausea Vomiting Diarrhoea		Lactic acidosis Weight loss		
Oral contra-ceptives	Nausea Vomiting Gastro- intestinal discomfort	Venous thrombo- embolism Myocardial infarction Stroke Subarachoid haemorrhage Oedema Hypertension	Weight gain Breast tenderness Cervical erosion Hyperglycaemia Altered libido Amenorrhoea Breakthrough bleeding Galactorrhoea	Dry eyes Intolerance to contact lenses Retinopathy	
Stanozolol	Stomatitis	Oedema	Amenorrhoea Weight gain Hypercalcaemia Azospermia Virilism (females)		
Thyroxine	Diarrhoea Vomiting	Tachycardia Angina Arrhythmias	Weight loss		

Immunological	Nervous	Renal/Hepatic	Skin/Joint	Other	Drug
	Lassitude		Rash	Weakness	**Metformin**

Angioneurotic oedema	Depression
	Headache
	Mood changes
		Hepatotoxicity
		Hepato-cellular
		  adenoma
		Gallstones
			Chloasma
			Skin and hair
			  changes
			Photosensitiv-
			  ity
				Increased
				  triglycerides
					**Oral
					contraceptives**

Angioneurotic oedema	Headache Euphoria Depression	Jaundice	Rash	Muscle cramps	**Stanozolol**
	Restlessness Insomnia Tremor Excitability Headache		Sweating	Fever	**Thyroxine**

5

Side-Effects of Drugs

Gastrointestinal drugs

Drug	Alimentary	Cardiovascular	Endocrine	Eye/ENT	Haematological
Bismuth chelate	Gastric irritation Anorexia Black stools			Blue colouration of gums Stomatitis	
Carbenoxolone	Heartburn	Oedema Hypertension	Sodium and water retention Alkalosis Hypokalaemia Impaired glucose tolerance		
Cholestyramine	Constipation Diarrhoea Heartburn Nausea Faecal impaction Steatorrhoea		Hyperchloraemic acidosis		
Cimetidine	Diarrhoea Acute pancreatitis	Cardiac arrhythmias Hypotension (rapid i.v.)	Gynaecomastia Loss of libido Hyperglycaemia Galactorrhoea Amenorrhoea	Laryngospasm	Bone marrow suppression Neutropenia Granulocytopenia Thrombocytopenia
Domperidone			Gynaecomastia		

Side-Effects of Drugs

mmunological	Nervous	Renal/Hepatic	Skin/Joint	Other	Drug

	Headache
	Malaise
	Confusion
	Tremor
	Impaired
	  coordination
		Hepatotoxicity
		Albuminuria
		Renal Failure
			Rash	Discolouration
				  of mucous
				  membranes
					**Bismuth
					  chelate**

		Renal failure
		Myoglobinuria
		Tubular
		  necrosis
		Changes in
		  liver function
			Rash	Myasthenia
				Myositis
				Muscle necrosis
					Carbenoxolone

			Skin rash Pruritus Osteoporosis		**Cholestyramine**

ngioneurotic
  oedema
	Dizziness
	Confusion
	Lightheaded-
	  ness
	Hallucinations
	Seizures
	Paranoia
	Motor
	  neuropathy
		Hepatotoxicity
		Interstitial
		  nephritis
			Rash
			Arthropathy
			Alopecia
			Urticaria
			Pruritus
			Exfoliative
			  dermatitis
				Muscle pain
				Myopathy
				Fever
					Cimetidine

	Extrapyramidal reactions				**Domperidone**

5

Side-Effects of Drugs

Gastrointestinal drugs *(cont'd)*

Drug	Alimentary	Cardiovascular	Endocrine	Eye/ENT	Haematological
Dicyclomine (also **Propantheline**)	Dry mouth Constipation Vomiting Retrosternal pain	Bradycardia Tachycardia Palpitations Postural hypotension Cardiac arrhythmias Precipitation of angina	Thirst	Dilation of pupils Photophobia Diplopia Glaucoma	
Loperamide	Abdominal pain Dry mouth Constipation				
Metoclopramide	Bowel disturbance		Gynaecomastia Galactorrhoea		
Pirenzepine	Dry mouth			Visual disturbance	
Ranitidine	Diarrhoea		Gynaecomastia		
Sucralfate	Constipation Epigastric pain				
Sulphasalazine	Vomiting Diarrhoea Metallic taste Pancreatitis	Raynaud's	Oligospermia Infertility		Agranulocytosis Haemolytic anaemia Megaloblastic anaemia Folate deficiency Lymphadeno-pathy
Ursodeoxy-cholic acid (also **Chenodeoxy-cholic acid**)	Diarrhoea Steatorrhoea				

Side-Effects of Drugs

Immunological	Nervous	Renal/Hepatic	Skin/Joint	Other	Drug
	Giddiness Staggering Restlessness Confusion Excitement Hallucinations Delirium Psychosis	Urinary retention	Flushing Dry skin Rash Eczema	Hyperpyrexia Rapid respiration	**Dicyclomine** (also **Propantheline**)
	Dizziness Headache		Rash	Fatigue	**Loperamide**
	Extrapyramidal effects Fatigue Drowsiness Lassitude Dizziness Faintness Restlessness Anxiety				**Metoclopramide**
					Pirenzepine
	Headache Dizziness	Raised liver enzymes	Rash		**Ranitidine**
					Sucralfate
Allergy Drug fever Anaphylaxis SLE		Hepatotoxicity	Rash Epidermal necrolysis Yellow pigmentation Stevens- Johnson	Pulmonary infiltration	**Sulpha- salazine**
		Raised liver enzymes	Pruritus		**Ursodeoxy- cholic acid** (also **Chenodeoxy- cholic acid**)

5

Side-Effects of Drugs

Drug	Alimentary	Cardiovascular	Endocrine	Eye/ENT	Haematological

Amantadine	Nausea
	Anorexia
	Vomiting
	Dry mouth
	Constipation
		Ankle oedema
		Orthostatic
		  hypotension
		Cardiac failure
				Visual
				  disturbance
					Leucopenia

Benzhexol	Dry mouth Thirst Vomiting Constipation	Bradycardia Tachycardia		Pupillary dilatation Glaucoma	

Benzodiaze-
pines
e.g.
Diazepam
Nitrazepam
	Nausea
	Constipation
	Altered
	  salivation
		Hypotension
		Thrombophleb-
		  itis (i.v.)
				Diplopia
				Vertigo
					Blood
					  dyscrasias

Butyrophen-
ones
e.g.
Haloperidol
	Dry mouth
	Constipation
		Postural
		  hypotension
		Tachycardia
		Arrhythmias
			Amenorrhoea
			Galactorrhoea
			Gynaecomastia
			Weight gain
			Hyperglycaemia
				Nasal
				  congestion
				Miosis
				Cataracts
				Corneal
				  opacities
					Blood
					  dyscrasias

Carbamazepine	Nausea	Fluid
		  retention
			Hyponatraemia		Aplastic
					  anaemia
					Agranulocytosis

Chloral
  hydrate
	Unpleasant
	  taste
	Gastric
	  irritation
	Vomiting
		Arrhythmias			Eosinophilia
					Leucopenia

Immunological	Nervous	Renal/Hepatic	Skin/Joint	Other	Drug

	Excitement
	Confusion
	Dizziness
	Slurred
	  speech
	Ataxia
	Depression
	Insomnia
	Tremor
	Psychosis
		Urinary
		  retention
			Livido
			  reticularis
			Rash
					Amantadine

	Giddiness Restlessness Confusion Excitement Hallucinations Psychosis	Desire to urinate	Flushing Rash		**Benzhexol**

	Drowsiness
	Ataxia
	Amnesia
	Dysarthria
	Depression
	Tremor
	Headache
	Dependence
		Urinary
		  retention
		Hepatotoxicity
			Rash	Respiratory
				  depression
				Altered
				  libido
					**Benzodiaze-
					pines**
					e.g.
					**Diazepam
					Nitrazepam**

SLE	Parkinsonism
	Drowsiness
	Agitation
	Insomnia
	Depression
	Convulsions
	Tardive
	  dyskinesia
		Jaundice
		Urinary
		  retention
			Photosensitiv-
			  ity
			Rash
			Urticaria
			Exfoliation
				Hypothermia
				Failure of
				  ejaculation
					**Butyrophen-
					ones**
					e.g.
					Haloperidol

SLE	Asthenia
	Drowsiness
	Diplopia
	Dizziness
	Headache
	Ataxia
		Oliguria
		Hepatotoxicity
			Rash
			Stevens-
			  Johnson
			Exfoliation
			Photosensitiv-
			  ity
					**Carbamaze-
					pine**

	Lightheaded- ness Ataxia Nightmares Excitement Confusion	Jaundice	Rash		**Chloral hydrate**

5

Side-Effects of Drugs

Drug	Alimentary	Cardiovascular	Endocrine	Eye/ENT	Haematological
Chlormethia-zole	Nausea Dyspepsia Vomiting	Hypotension Thrombophle- bitis (i.v.)		Sneezing Conjunctivitis	
Ethosuximide	Anorexia Nausea Vomiting Hiccough			Photophobia	Eosinophilia Blood dyscrasias
Fenfluramine	Nausea Diarrhoea Dry mouth Flatulence Dyspepsia Constipation	Palpitations Fluid retention	Impotence		Haemolytic anaemia
Levodopa	Anorexia Nausea Vomiting Abdominal pain Constipation Diarrhoea Dysphagia Dyspepsia GI bleeding	Postural hypotension Palpitations Flushing Arrhythmias Hypertension	Priapism	Miosis Mydriasis Diplopia Glaucoma	Leucopenia Haemolytic anaemia
Lithium	Nausea Diarrhoea Dyspepsia Dry mouth Constipation Metallic taste	Oedema Arrhythmias	Thirst Weight gain Hypothyroidism Hyperthyroid- ism	Blurred vision Stuffy nose	Leucocytosis

5

Side-Effects of Drugs

Immunological	Nervous	Renal/Hepatic	Skin/Joint	Other	Drug
	Drowsiness Dependence	Hepatotoxicity		Bronchial irritation	**Chlormethia- zole**

SLE	Drowsiness
	Lethargy
	Euphoria
	Headache
	Dizziness
	Agitation
	Aggression
	Extrapyramidal
	  reactions
			Rash
			Urticaria
			Stevens-
			  Johnson
					Ethosuximide

	Headache Dizziness Sedation Insomnia Depression Nightmares Euphoria Dependence	Urinary frequency	Rash Alopecia	Fatigue	**Fenfluramine**

	Faintness
	Dizziness
	Agitation
	Anxiety
	Elation
	Insomnia
	Drowsiness
	Depression
	Aggression
	Hallucinations
	Delusions
	Involuntary
	  movements
	Headache
	Peripheral
	  neuropathy
		Polyuria
		Incontinence
		Difficulty in
		  micturition
		Abnormal liver
		  function
		Azotaemia
			Rash
			Hair fall
				Sweating
				Muscle
				  twitching
				Hoarseness
					Levodopa

	Tremor
	Apathy
	Drowsiness
	Lethargy
	Headache
	Ataxia
	Dysarthria
	Convulsions
	Rigidity
	Coma
		Polyuria
		Nephrogenic
		  diabetes
		  insipidus
			Grey
			  colouration
			Acne
			Psoriasis
			Flushing
				Weakness
				Twitching
				Aching
					Lithium

5

Side-Effects of Drugs

Drug	Alimentary	Cardiovascular	Endocrine	Eye/ENT	Haematological
Mazindol	Dry mouth Metallic taste Anorexia Nausea Constipation Diarrhoea	Hypertension Tachycardia Angina Arrhythmias	Altered libido	Mydriasis	Aplastic anaemia
Meprobamate	Nausea Vomiting Diarrhoea	Hypotension Tachycardia Arrhythmias		Disturbed vision	Blood dyscrasias
Mianserin		Postural hypotension	Weight gain Hyperglycaemia		Agranulocyto- sis
Monoamine oxidase inhibitors e.g. **Phenelzine**	Dry mouth Constipation Nausea Vomiting	Postural hypotension Oedema Hypertensive crisis	Sexual disturbance Bulimia	Blurred vision	Aplastic anaemia Leucopenia
Nomifensine	Nausea Dry mouth	Tachycardia			Haemolytic anaemia

Immunological	Nervous	Renal/Hepatic	Skin/Joint	Other	Drug
	Agitation Insomnia Restlessness Headache Tremor Psychosis Dependence Depression				**Mazindol**
Angioneurotic oedema Bronchospasm	Drowsiness Paraesthesiae Headache Excitement Dizziness Ataxia Dependence	Anuria	Rash Urticaria Purpura Erythema multiforme	Weakness	**Meprobamate**
	Drowsiness Mania		Rash		**Mianserin**

	Dizziness
	Drowsiness
	Agitation
	Tremor
	Insomnia
	Confusion
	Convulsions
	Hallucinations
	Psychosis
	Hypomania
	Peripheral
	  neuropathy
		Difficulty with
		  micturition
		Hepatotoxicity
			Rash	Fatigue	**Monoamine
					oxidase
					inhibitors**
					e.g.
					Phenelzine

	Restlessness Insomnia Headache Dizziness Nightmares Paranoid delusions Drowsiness			Fever	**Nomifensine**

Side-Effects of Drugs

5

Drug	Alimentary	Cardiovascular	Endocrine	Eye/ENT	Haematological
Orphenadrine	Dry mouth Constipation Vomiting	Tachycardia Arrhythmias Hypertension	Thirst	Dilated pupils Photophobia Glaucoma	
Phenobarbi- tone				Nystagmus	Megaloblastic anaemia
Phenothi- azines e.g. **Chlorprom- azine**	Dry mouth Constipation	Postural hypotension Tachycardia Arrhythmias	Inhibition of ejaculation Amenorrhoea Galactorrhoea Gynaecomastia Weight gain Hyperglycaemia	Nasal congestion Miosis Mydriasis Corneal and lens opacities	Agranulocyto- sis Haemolytic anaemia Eosinophilia
Phenytoin	Nausea Vomiting Anorexia Dyspepsia Gum hyper- trophy		Hyperglycaemia	Nystagmus Diplopia	Megaloblastic anaemia Blood dyscrasias
Primidone	Nausea Vomiting			Vertigo Diplopia Nystagmus	Megaloblastic anaemia Leucopenia Thrombocyto- penia
Selegeline	Nausea	Hypotension			

nmunological	Nervous	Renal/Hepatic	Skin/Joint	Other	Drug
	Giddiness Staggering Sedation Confusion Excitement Hallucinations	Urinary retention	Flushing Rash	Pyrexia Hyperven- tilation	**Orphenadrine**
	Sedation Ataxia Irritability Hyperactivity (children) Confusion Dependence	Hepatotoxicity	Rash Exfoliation Purpura Stevens- Johnson	Osteomalacia Teratogenicity	**Phenobarbitone**
LE	Drowsiness Agitation Insomnia Depression Convulsions Parkinsonism Tardive dyskinesia	Hepatotoxicity Urinary retention	Photosensitivity Rash Urticaria Exfoliation Pigmentation	Hypothermia Hyperpyrexia	**Phenothi- azines** e.g. **Chlorprom- azine**
LE ymphadeno- pathy educed IgA seudo lymphoma	Headache Tremor Ataxia Dysarthria Aggression Depression Peripheral neuropathy Encephalopathy Cerebellar degeneration Paradoxical seizures	Hepatotoxicity	Rash Acne Hirsutism Coarse facies Stevens- Johnson Dupytren's contracture	Osteomalacia Teratogenicity Lymphoma	**Phenytoin**
LE ymphadeno- pathy	Sedation Dizziness Ataxia Psychosis		Rash	Osteomalacia	**Primidone**
	Confusion Psychosis				**Selegeline**

Psychoactive drugs *(cont'd)*

Drug	Alimentary	Cardiovascular	Endocrine	Eye/ENT	Haematological
Sodium valproate	Anorexia Nausea Vomiting Pancreatitis	Oedema	Weight gain		Thrombocyto- penia Neutropenia
Sulthiame	Anorexia Nausea Weight loss Abdominal pain Vomiting			Ptosis	Leucopenia

Trazodone	Nausea
	Vomiting
	Dry mouth
	Constipation
	Diarrhoea
		Bradycardia
		Tachycardia
		Postural
		  hypotension
			Weight gain
			Priapism
				Blurred
				  vision	

Tricyclic anti-depressants e.g. **Amitripty-line Imipramine**	Dry mouth
	Metallic taste
	Constipation
	Nausea
	Vomiting
	Weight loss
		Tachycardia
		Postural
		  hypotension
		Hypertension
		Arrhythmias
			Weight gain
			Bulimia
			Altered libido
			Impotence
			Gynaecomastia
			Inappropriate
			  ADH
				Blurred
				  vision
				Glaucoma
					Blood
					  dyscrasias

Tryptophan	Nausea Anorexia				
Viloxazine	Nausea Vomiting Dry mouth Constipation	Tachycardia Hypertension			

Side-Effects of Drugs

5

Immunological	Nervous	Renal/Hepatic	Skin/Joint	Other	Drug
	Drowsiness Tremor Confusion Irritability Ataxia	Hepatotoxicity	Rash Alopecia	Teratogenicity	**Sodium valproate**
	Paraesthesiae Drowsiness Ataxia Headache Depression Psychosis Insomnia		Rash	Dyspnoea	**Sulthiame**
	Drowsiness Dizziness Headache Tremor Restlessness Confusion Insomnia		Rash	Weakness	**Trazodone**
	Drowsiness Tremor Dizziness Ataxia Seizures Extrapyramidal symptoms Hypomania Delirium	Urinary retention Hepatotoxicity	Rash Photosensitivity	Sweating Fatigue	**Tricyclic anti-depressants** e.g. **Amitriptyline Imipramine**
	Drowsiness				**Tryptophan**
	Headache Anxiety Agitation Drowsiness Confusion Ataxia Dizziness Insomnia Nightmares Tremor Paraesthesiae Convulsions	Difficulty with micturition Jaundice	Rash	Muscle pain Sweating	**Viloxazine**

Other Drugs

Drug	Alimentary	Cardiovascular	Endocrine	Eye/ENT	Haematological
Acyclovir					Mild anaemia
Antihistamines e.g. **Promethazine Chlorpheniram-ine**	Anorexia Nausea Vomiting Epigastric pain Diarrhoea Constipation Dry mouth	Hypotension		Blurred vision Tinnitus	Agranulocytosis Haemolytic anaemia
Baclofen	Nausea Vomiting Diarrhoea Constipation	Hypotension		Visual disturbance	
Beta agonists e.g. **Salbutamol Terbutaline**		Palpitations Hypotension			
Chloroquine	Nausea Vomiting Diarrhoea Abdominal cramps	Hypotension Cardiovascular collapse		Diplopia Corneal opacities Macular lesions Optic atrophy Blindness Tinnitus Deafness	Blood dyscrasias
Cromoglycate	Nausea Vomiting			Nasal congestion	

Side-Effects of Drugs

Immunological	Nervous	Renal/Hepatic	Skin/Joint	Other	Drug
	Neurological reactions	Reversible renal impairment Raised liver enzymes	Rash		**Acyclovir**
	Sedation Dizziness Incoordination Headache Depression Elation Nightmares Seizures Dyskinesia	Difficulty with micturition Hepatotoxicity	Rash Eczema	Weakness	**Antihistamines** e.g. **Promethazine Chlorpheniram- ine**
	Drowsiness Confusion Dizziness Euphoria Hallucinations Insomnia Depression Headache Tremor	Hepatotoxicity Urinary disturbance	Rash Pruritus	Fatigue Hypotonia	**Baclofen**
	Tremor Headaches Tension			Muscle cramps	**Beta agonists** e.g. **Salbutamol Terbutaline**
	Headache Convulsions Psychosis		Rash Purpura Pruritus Urticaria Alopecia Pigmentation Photosensi- tivity	Myopathy	**Chloroquine**
Angioneurotic oedema Anaphylaxis	Headache Dizziness		Rash Urticaria Arthralgia	Wheezing Cough Bronchospasm	**Cromoglycate**

Side-Effects of Drugs

Drug	Alimentary	Cardiovascular	Endocrine	Eye/ENT	Haematological
Dantrolene	Diarrhoea Dysphagia				
Emepromium bromide	Oesophageal ulceration Buccal ulceration Dry mouth Constipation Vomiting	Tachycardia		Glaucoma	
Ephedrine	Nausea Vomiting	Tachycardia Chest pain Palpitations Hypertension Arrhythmias			
Griseofulvin	Dry mouth Altered taste GI disturbance				Leucopenia
Ketoconazole	Nausea Vomiting		Gynaecomastia		
Ketotifen	Dry mouth		Weight gain Increased appetite		
Nabilone	Dry mouth Abdominal cramps	Tachycardia Postural hypotension	Decreased appetite	Blurred vision	
Quinine	Nausea Abdominal pain			Tinnitus Disturbed vision Temporary blindness	Haemolytic anaemia Thrombocyto- penia
Theophylline	Nausea Vomiting GI bleeding	Palpitations Hypotension		Visual disorder Vertigo	

Immunological	Nervous	Renal/Hepatic	Skin/Joint	Other	Drug
	Drowsiness Dizziness Convulsions	Hepatotoxicity	Rash Pruritus	Weakness Malaise	**Dantrolene**
	Giddiness		Rash		**Emepromium bromide**
	Giddiness Headache Tremor Anxiety Insomnia Hallucinations Psychosis Seizures	Difficulty with micturition		Sweating Weakness	**Ephedrine**

gioneurotic
oedema
E
	Headache
	Paraesthesiae
	Confusion
	Irritability
	Depression
		Proteinuria
		Hepatitis
			Rash
			Erythema
			  multiforme
			Exfoliation
			Photosensitiv-
			  ity
				Fatigue	**Griseofulvin**

	Headache Dizziness	Hepatitis	Rash Pruritus	Teratogenicity	**Ketoconazole**
	Drowsiness Ataxia				**Ketotifen**
	Euphoria Drowsiness Dizziness Headache Ataxia Impaired concentration Depression Hallucinations Psychosis Tremor				**Nabilone**
gioneurotic oedema	Headache		Rash Pruritus Stevens- Johnson		**Quinine**
	Headache Insomnia Confusion Agitation Convulsions			Hyperventila- tion	**Theophylline**

Side-Effects of Drugs

6

Drug Interactions

INTRODUCTION

With the increasing use of chronic drug therapy, the introduction of more potent therapeutic agents coupled with better understanding of drug action and greater access to drug assays, the potential for and recognition of adverse drug interactions is increasing. Many interactions are unpredictable and, therefore, unavoidable. Many more are eminently predictable. Although there are too many interactions to keep easily in mind, only a few have important repercussions for the patient. These are confined to drugs with a narrow therapeutic index and often occur in well-defined clinical situations.

Drugs at risk of interaction

Only a small number of drugs are consistently implicated in adverse drug interactions. They may affect a vital process such as clotting, respiration, cardiac rhythm or glucose homeostasis or have a steep dose-response curve, such that an increase in dose will produce a similar increment in response, e.g. antihypertensives, tranquillisers, opiates and calcium antagonists. Some drugs show major concentration-dependent toxicity, e.g. aminoglycoside antibiotics, lithium, theophylline, digoxin, warfarin and methotrexate whereas for others loss of pharmacological effect may be of equal or greater clinical importance, e.g. corticosteroids, phenytoin, quinidine, oral contraceptives, chlorpromazine and rifampicin. Phenytoin is uniquely susceptible to inhibitory drug interactions as its hepatic metabolism is saturable. Many of these drugs have in common a narrow therapeutic index. A small increase in plasma concentration may produce toxicity whereas a small decrease may result in loss of therapeutic effect. They are often potent therapeutic agents which are in widespread clinical use.

Patients at risk of interaction

Particular patient populations may be at increased risk both of sustaining a drug interaction and suffering severe clinical repercussions therefrom. Most severely ill patients receive a number of drugs and it may be difficult to dissect out iatrogenic toxicity from the underlying clinical presentation. Patients with cardiac failure, aplastic anaemia or hepatic pre-coma may have little leeway for further deterioration following the development of a new clinical problem. Cardiac arrhythmias, severe epilepsy, brittle diabetes or status asthmaticus may be further exacerbated by an adverse interaction which may have minor consequences in another less vulnerable patient. Loss of therapeutic effect may be particularly relevant where a potentially dangerous pathological process is being suppressed such as malignancy, connective tissue disorder or Addison's disease. The presence of hypoxia or hypothyroidism may increase the susceptibility of the patient to adverse effects from a drug combination which was previously well tolerated. Disease affecting the major organs responsible for eliminating drug from the body may increase the likelihood of an interaction. Patients with

Drug Interactions

severe parenchymatous liver disease or chronic renal failure clearly fall into this category. The effect of hepatic anoxia or congestion on drug metabolism in cardiac failure is often overlooked. An intercurrent viral hepatitis or pneumonic illness may alter drug elimination or response. A minor deterioration in glomerular filtration rate may produce increasing nephrotoxicity if the patient is receiving drugs which themselves cause renal damage either singly or in combination, e.g. frusemide and gentamicin, bendrofluazide and lithium. Finally, the biggest risk group is the elderly who often receive polypharmacy. They are particularly susceptible to adverse effects especially involving the central nervous system. In addition, comprehension may be poor and so dosage regimens must be kept simple. Thus when a patient's clinical condition changes, particularly if he is severely ill or elderly, all his medication should be reviewed.

Mechanisms of interactions

The problems of remembering all the clinically important interactions can be offset by considering the major mechanisms involved. This will also help in predicting problems and recognising new interactions. Such an understanding will also allow the correct clinical decision to be made. Adverse drug interactions can be conveniently divided into those involving the pharmacokinetics of the drug and those affecting the pharmacodynamic response to the drug. Pharmacokinetic interactions may affect absorption, distribution or elimination processes. Because of the marked interindividual variation in these events, such interactions may be expected but their extent cannot be predicted. In only a few will there be serious clinical consequences. Pharmacodynamic effects are less easily classified but are in the main, more predictable, and may provide fascinating insights into the mode of action of a drug or the pathophysiology of a disease state.

Absorption

If drug absorption is reduced, its concentration at the site of action is also reduced. Antacids containing divalent and trivalent cations form insoluble complexes with some drugs such as tetracycline, iron and prednisolone. The anion exchange resin, cholestyramine binds acidic drugs such as digoxin and warfarin as well as bile salts. Kaolin-pectin mixtures can also adsorb drugs. These interactions depend on the simultaneous presence of both drugs in the stomach and can be avoided by separating the doses by 2 hours. As drugs are absorbed optimally in the upper small bowel, delayed gastric emptying will reduce the time to and extent of the peak plasma level of a drug. The bioavailability is only changed if the drug is also biodegraded within the gastric lumen or wall as is the case with chlorpromazine, levodopa and pivampicillin. This type of interaction has most clinical relevance if a rapid, high peak concentration of the drug is important, e.g. analgesics and antibiotics. There are a large number of drug groups which themselves slow gastric emptying including anticholinergics, tricyclic antidepressants, antihistamines, phenothiazines and opiates. Metoclopramide may accelerate gastric emptying and, therefore, drug absorption. Drugs which cause local mucosal damage (neomycin, colchicine, cytotoxic agents) can reduce the absorption of other poorly-absorbed substances, e.g. phenytoin, digoxin.

There are several potentially important interactions involving changes in gastrointestinal flora produced by the major groups of broad spectrum antibiotics. A small number of women taking an oral contraceptive agent may be put at risk of pregnancy by the prescription of a broad spectrum antibiotic for a minor infection. The mechanism is thought to involve disruption of the enterohepatic cycling of the hormonal components by removal of the gut bacteria responsible for their deconjugation. An additional method of contraception may be advised during this time. Antibiotics have also been shown to reduce the bacterial inactivation of digoxin in the gut lumen increasing, occasionally substantially, its bioavailability. This may produce digoxin toxicity in a susceptible patient.

Enzyme induction

A variety of drugs bind to intracellular receptors in a number of organs, the liver being the most important, to activate the production of monooxygenase and some conjugative enzymes. As protein synthesis is required, the maximum effect is not seen for 2–3 weeks. The clinical result is increased metabolism of a number of drugs eliminated by the liver with concomitant attenuation of their pharmacological effects. The most potent enzyme inducers in clinical use are the antibiotic, rifampicin and the anticonvulsants, phenobarbitone, phenytoin and carbamazepine. Primidone is metabolised in part to phenobarbitone and sulphinpyrazone can induce the metabolism of some drugs and inhibit others. Drugs showing loss of effect with concurrent enzyme inducers include corticosteroids, oral contraceptives, warfarin, quinidine and opiates. These all produce important clinical effects and demand increased dosage of the induced drug. Conversely when the inducing agent is withdrawn, the process goes into reverse with reduction in the number of enzymes resulting in a gradual increase in the plasma level of the interacted drug which may result in toxicity. As most drugs are inactivated in the liver, this mechanism will be implicated in many interactions.

Enzyme inhibition

Drugs which are biotransformed in the liver can have their metabolism inhibited, usually competitively. This produces an increase in plasma level of the inhibited drug which is maximal five half-lives later, i.e. a new steady state is produced. Potentiation of its pharmacological effects can, therefore, occur very quickly for some drugs with a short half-life, e.g. sulphonylureas or over a week with others which are eliminated more slowly, e.g. diazepam, warfarin. When an inhibition interaction is recognised the inhibitor can be discontinued or the dose of the target drug reduced. Many commonly used drugs have inhibitory properties including allopurinol, cimetidine,

Drug Interactions

sodium valproate, dextropropoxyphene (in Distalgesic), oral contraceptives and some tricyclic antidepressants and phenothiazines. The antibiotics erythromycin, metronidazole and a number of the sulphonamides including sulphamethoxazole (in co-trimoxazole) are particularly dangerous as they are introduced in a short course in patients who are often already receiving a number of other drugs. The most clinically relevant of such interactions involve drugs with a narrow therapeutic ratio, e.g. warfarin, phenytoin, theophylline. A number of fatal inhibitory interactions are reported with warfarin each year.

Not all inhibitory interactions concern hepatic enzymes. Allopurinol, a xanthine oxidase inhibitor, potentiates the actions of 6-mercaptopurine and azathioprine which are metabolised in part by xanthine oxidase. When an inhibiting drug is withdrawn the plasma concentration of the target drug will fall with some reduction in its therapeutic effect. Inhibitory interactions are particularly perfidious because the extent of the effect is so unpredictable.

First pass metabolism

Any drug which inhibits hepatic monooxygenase activity may increase the bioavailability of oxidised drugs with a substantial first pass metabolism such as verapamil, chlorpromazine and amitriptyline. The most important interactions are produced by cimetidine and propranolol. Conversely enzyme inducers accelerate drug metabolism and will reduce the bioavailability of these drugs. There is some evidence that some drugs with high first pass metabolism given in combination may compete for metabolic enzyme sites. They may augment each other's bioavailability and mutually inhibit one another's metabolism, e.g. chlorpromazine and propranolol.

Non-selective monoamine oxidase (MAO) inhibitors, such as phenelzine and tranylcypromine, directly inhibit the first pass metabolism of tyramine (in cheese, tomatoes, chocolate, bananas, yeast products, red wine, etc.) and phenylpropanolamine and pseudoephedrine in proprietary cough mixtures. Substantial amounts of these amines reach the sympathetic nervous system and stimulate the release of intraneuronal noradrenaline. Inhibition of intrasynaptic MAO further increases noradrenaline effects producing a syndrome of sympathetic overactivity characterised by severe hypertension, excitement, hyperpyrexia and delirium which may result in a subarachnoid haemorrhage. As MAO is inhibited irreversibly, this interaction can occur for up to 2 weeks after the antidepressant has been discontinued.

Protein binding displacement

When one drug is displaced by another from its binding sites on plasma proteins, there is a transient rise in free concentration which, almost instantaneously, is distributed throughout the tissues. A compensatory increase in metabolism or excretion occurs such that a new steady state free concentration is produced similar to that present before the displacing drug was added. The total drug level falls to accommodate the rise in free fraction (percentage free/total concentration). The pharmacological effect produced is minimal. The overemphasis in the clinical importance of this type of interaction comes from situations where protein binding displacement is also accompanied by enzyme inhibition, e.g. phenylbutazone potentiation of warfarin anticoagulation, sodium valproate potentiation of phenytoin toxicity. A protein binding displacement interaction will only otherwise be noticeable clinically if the displaced drug is bound in tissues, e.g. sulphonamide displacement of bilirubin in premature infants to produce kernicterus or if the displaced drug has a small distribution volume, a narrow therapeutic ratio and a very rapid onset of action, e.g. methotrexate.

Renal excretion

Interference with the renal excretion of a drug is only important if the fraction excreted unchanged is large, i.e. the drug is water soluble. Once again a narrow therapeutic ratio is required for toxicity to be produced. The best examples occur with digoxin and lithium. Amiodarone, quinidine, quinine and verapamil all significantly reduce renal digoxin elimination, substantially increasing serum digoxin concentration. Thiazide and 'loop' diuretics and non-steroidal anti-inflammatory agents reduce lithium excretion and may potentiate its neuro- and nephrotoxicity. Any reduction in its clearance may thus become self increasing. As aminoglycoside antibiotics are primarily filtered by the kidney, any drug which reduces glomerular filtration rate will also reduce aminoglycoside excretion. Therapeutic drug monitoring of digoxin, lithium and the aminoglycosides may help to avoid or recognise such drug interactions.

Weak acids and bases are excreted by separate active tubular transport systems. These drugs will compete for such excretory pathways and this is the basis for the well-known effect of probenecid in increasing penicillin and cephalosporin levels. However, probenecid also increases methotrexate toxicity and phenylbutazone enhances the hypoglycaemic effect of chlorpropamide by the same mechanism. Competition for these active transport systems can be expected to occur to a variable extent with all weakly acidic and basic drugs. This may be the way cimetidine reduces procainamide elimination.

Synergism

The commonest type of drug interaction in clinical medicine probably involves synergism between two drugs acting on the same system, organ, cell or enzyme. Such an interaction may be clinically useful as with the components of the oral contraceptive pill and of co-trimoxazole. Thus all drugs which have a depressant function on the central nervous system, e.g. ethanol, benzodiazepines, tricyclic antidepressants, antihistamines, phenothiazines, methyldopa and clonidine will potentiate one another's sedative action. All non-steroidal anti-inflammatory agents reduce platelet adhesiveness thereby potentiating warfarin anticoagulation. They may also provide a site of bleeding in the stomach. These effects are not related to protein-binding displacement which is often blamed. Aminoglycosides potentiate the muscle relaxant effects of ganglion-blocking drugs in anaesthesia. The calcium antagonist verapamil may produce severe bradycardia or atrio-ventricular block in a patient already receiving digoxin. In a similar way calcium antagonists and beta blockers, both of which have negative inotropic actions, may precipitate cardiac failure in a susceptible patient.

Antagonism

Drugs acting on the same cellular mechanism may also antagonise one another's pharmacological effects. Some such antagonisms are obvious and easily avoided, e.g. beta agonists and blockers, vitamin K and warfarin, thiazide diuretics and hypoglycaemic agents. Others are less easily predicted, e.g. the abolition of the ulcer healing effect of carbenoxolone by spironolactone, antagonism of the antihypertensive effect of the presynaptic alpha agonist clonidine by imipramine which has weak alpha blocking properties. Other unexpected examples may give fascinating insights into the mode of drug action. Thus the reversal of the blood pressure lowering effects of thiazides and beta-blockers by non-steroidal anti-inflammatory drugs suggests a local renal prostaglandin mediated mode of action for these antihypertensive agents. These observations have important implications for the management of hypertension in patients with rheumatoid disease and osteoarthrosis.

Cellular transport systems

A number of drugs enter the cell by utilising a physiological transport system. The adrenergic neurone blocking drugs, bethanidine, debrisoquine and guanethidine, are concentrated over 1000 fold from the plasma to the adrenergic nerve ending by the 'amine pump'. Inhibition of this pump by the tricyclic antidepressants or high dose neuroleptics will antagonise their antihypertensive effect by inhibiting this transport system, thus reducing the concentration of these drugs at the nerve ending. Pizotifen and mazindol appear to interact with adrenergic neurone blocking drugs by the same mechanism. Indirectly acting sympathetic amines such as ephedrine, phenylephrine, and phenylpropanolamine also compete for amine uptake and storage processes. Since these are common ingredients of proprietary cough and cold preparations, patients receiving adrenergic neurone blocking agents should be specifically warned of this possible interaction.

Indirect receptor effects

Drug combinations may produce interactions by an interplay of receptor effects. Non-selective beta blockers such as propranolol may prolong the duration of hypoglycaemia by inhibiting the compensatory breakdown of glycogen in a diabetic patient zealously treated with insulin or a sulphonylurea. This inhibition of tissue glycogenolysis is mediated by β_2 receptors and so more cardio-selective agents such as atenolol and metoprolol are less likely to do this. All these drugs, however, will mask the sympathetically-mediated warning signs of hypoglycaemia such as tachycardia, tremor and sweating and this is the more important adverse interaction in this clinical setting. An indirect receptor interaction may be responsible for the neurotoxicity (lethargy, confusion, forgetfulness, dysphoria, ataxia) reported in lithium-treated patients receiving concurrent neuroleptics or carbamazepine as the serum lithium concentration is unaltered. Although uncommon, this is an important interaction as these drugs are often used in combination in the acutely disturbed manic patient.

Fluid and electrolyte imbalance

Diuretics may be involved in drug interactions in a number of ways. Digoxin and potassium ions compete for the same binding sites on Na/K ATPase and this explains the potentiation of digoxin toxicity by hypokalaemia produced by concomitant diuretic therapy. Severely hypokalaemic patients may exhibit toxicity at serum digoxin concentrations within the 'therapeutic range' of 0.8–2 ng/ml (1–2.6 nmol/l). By decreasing sodium reabsorption in the proximal tubule, lithium reabsorption is increased leading to a dose-dependent rise in serum lithium concentration. Loop diuretics may produce increased tissue concentrations of nephrotoxic drug such as gentamicin in the renal tubule. Treatment of congestive cardiac failure may improve hepatic drug metabolising capacity and blood flow, thereby hastening the elimination of lipid soluble drugs.

Conclusions

Drug interactions are ubiquitous but only rarely produce major adverse repercussions for the patient. It is this individual variation in outcome produced by combinations of drugs which causes the major difficulty. Thus one patient may show little or no adverse effect whereas another may manifest a catastrophic life-threatening interaction. The background genetic and environmental factors involved clearly are important influences and whenever possible these should be considered *before* adding or withdrawing therapy. There follows a list of the most clinically relevant drug interactions together with some indication of the mechanism responsible and the possible outcome. Such a list cannot be completely comprehensive as hardly a month passes without the description of a new interaction in the journals. These can often be anticipated by considering the pharmacological effects and pharmacokinetic features of the drugs concerned.

	Interacting drug	Mechanism	Possible outcome
Acetazolamide	Lithium	Increased renal excretion	Reduced lithium effect
	Mexiletine	Decreased excretion	Increased circulating mexilitine
	Quinidine	Decreased excretion	Increased circulating quinidine
Acetohexamide	Phenylbutazone	Reduced excretion of active metabolite	Hypoglycaemia
Allopurinol	Azathioprine	Enzyme inhibition	Azathioprine toxicity
	Cyclophosphamide	Uncertain	Bone marrow toxicity
	Mercaptopurine	Enzyme inhibition	Mercaptopurine toxicity
	Phenytoin	Enzyme inhibition	Phenytoin toxicity
	Theophylline	Enzyme inhibition	Theophylline toxicity
	Warfarin	Enzyme inhibition	Potentiated anticoagulation
Amiloride	Carbenoxolone	Antagonism	Inhibition of ulcer healing
	Potassium supplements	Additive	Hyperkalaemia
Aminoglutethimide	Dexamethasone	Enzyme induction	Reduced steroid effect
	Warfarin	Enzyme induction	Reduced anticoagulation
Aminoglycosides	Cephaloridine	Synergism	Nephrotoxicity
	Ethacrynic acid	Additive	Ototoxicity, nephrotoxicity
	Frusemide	Reduced renal excretion	Ototoxicity, nephrotoxicity
	Neuromuscular blockers	Additive	Increased blockade
	Penicillins	Incompatibility in infusions	Treatment failure
	Polymixins	Additive	Nephrotoxicity
Amiodarone	Digoxin	Reduction in renal excretion	Digoxin toxicity
	Disopyramide	Synergism	Ventricular arrhythmias
	Quinidine	Enzyme inhibition	Quinidine toxicity
	Warfarin	Enzyme inhibition	Potentiated anticoagulation
Amphetamines	Monoamine oxidase inhibitors	Increased intrasynaptic amines	Severe hypertension
Amphotericin	Digoxin	Production of hypo-kalaemia	Digoxin toxicity
	Neuromuscular blockers	Production of hypo-kalaemia	Potentiation
Ampicillin	Atenolol	Reduced absorption	Possible reduced beta blockade
	Oral contraceptives	Reduced enterohepatic circulation	Contraceptive failure

6

Drug Interactions

	Interacting drug	Mechanism	Possible outcome
Anabolic steroids	Warfarin	Synergism	Potentiated anti-coagulation
Antacids	Aspirin	Complexes in gut lumen	Treatment failure
	Chlorpromazine	Complexes in gut lumen	Reduced chlorpromazine absorption
	Digoxin	Binding in gut lumen	Reduced digoxin effect
	Ethambutol	Reduced absorption	Treatment failure
	Iron	Insoluble complexes in gut lumen	Reduced iron absorption
	Isoniazid	Decreased absorption	Treatment failure
	Ketoconazole	Impaired absorption	Loss of ketoconazole effect
	Levodopa	Increasing gastric emptying	Enhanced levodopa absorption
	Penicillamine	Binding in gut lumen	Reduced penicillamine absorption
	Quinidine	Reduced tubular reabsorption	Increased renal quinidine excretion
	Tetracyclines	Insoluble complexes in gut lumen	Treatment failure
Anticholinergics	Chlorpromazine	Delayed gastric emptying	Reduced chlorpromazine bioavailability
	Digoxin	Delayed gastric emptying	Increased digoxin absorption
	Lithium	Delayed gastric emptying	Reduced lithium absorption
	Tricyclic anti-depressants	Synergism	Anticholinergic side-effects
Aspirin	Antacids	Complexes in gut lumen	Treatment failure
	Captopril	Unknown	Reduction in captopril effect
	Methotrexate	Competition for active renal transport	Methotrexate toxicity
	Probenecid	Antagonism	Loss of uricosuric effect
	Warfarin	Synergism	Haemorrhage
Atenolol	Ampicillin	Reduced absorption	Possible reduced beta blockade
	Insulin	Blocking cardiovascular response	Masking of hypoglycaemic symptoms
	Verapamil	Synergism	Cardiac failure, conduction defects
Azapropazone	Phenytoin	Enzyme inhibition	Phenytoin toxicity
	Tolbutamide	Enzyme inhibition	Hypoglycaemia
	Warfarin	Enzyme inhibition	Potentiated anti-coagulation
Azathioprine	Allopurinol	Enzyme inhibition	Azathioprine toxicity

6

Drug Interactions

	Interacting drug	Mechanism	Possible outcome
Bethanidine	Chlorpromazine	Inhibition of neuronal uptake	Reduced hypotension
	Ephedrine	Competition for neuronal uptake	Reduced hypotension
	Mazindol	Inhibition of neuronal uptake	Reduced hypotension
	Phenylephrine	Competition for neuronal uptake	Reduced hypotension
	Phenylpropanolamine	Competition for neuronal uptake	Reduced hypotension
	Pizotifen	Inhibition of neuronal uptake	Reduced hypotension
	Tricyclic anti-depressants	Inhibition of neuronal uptake	Reduced hypotension
Bumetanide	Digoxin	Production of hypo-kalaemia	Digoxin toxicity
	Indomethacin	Antagonism	Reduced diuresis
	Lithium	Increased tubular reabsorption	Lithium toxicity
Captopril	Aspirin	Unknown	Reduction in captopril effect
	Indomethacin	Unknown	Reduction in captopril effect
	Potassium supplements	Additive	Hyperkalaemia
Carbamazepine	Cimetidine	Enzyme inhibition	Carbamazepine toxicity
	Clonazepam	Enzyme induction	Reduced clonazepam concentration
	Dextropropoxyphene	Enzyme inhibition	Carbamazepine toxicity
	Erythromycin	Enzyme inhibition	Carbamazepine toxicity
	Ethosuximide	Enzyme induction	Decreased ethosuximide effect
	Isoniazid	Enzyme inhibition	Carbamazepine toxicity
	Lithium	Synergism	Lithium toxicity
	Oral contraceptives	Enzyme induction	Contraceptive failure
	Phenytoin	Mutual enzyme induction	Reduced concentration of both
	Sodium valproate	Enzyme induction	Reduced valproate concentration
	Theophylline	Enzyme induction	Reduced theophylline effect
	Warfarin	Enzyme induction	Reduced anticoagulation
Carbenoxolone	Amiloride	Antagonism	Inhibition of ulcer healing
	Spironolactone	Antagonism	Inhibition of ulcer healing

	Interacting drug	Mechanism	Possible outcome
Cephaloridine	Aminoglycosides	Synergism	Nephrotoxicity
	Ethacrynic acid	Increased intra-renal concentration	Nephrotoxicity
	Frusemide	Increased intra-renal concentration	Nephrotoxicity
Cephalosporins	Probenecid	Competition for active renal transport	Increased circulating cephalosporin
Chloral hydrate	Ethanol	Inhibition of acetaldehyde oxidation	Antabuse reaction
Chloramphenicol	Phenytoin	Enzyme inhibition	Phenytoin toxicity
	Tolbutamide	Enzyme inhibition	Hypoglycaemia
	Warfarin	Enzyme inhibition	Potentiated anticoagulation
Chlordiazepoxide	Cimetidine	Enzyme inhibition	Increased circulating chlordiazepoxide
	Disulfiram	Enzyme inhibition	Increased circulating chlordiazepoxide
	Ethanol	Enzyme inhibition	Increased circulating chlordiazepoxide
	Oral contraceptives	Enzyme inhibition	Increased circulating chlordiazepoxide
Chlormethiazole	Cimetidine	Enzyme inhibition	Chlormethiazole toxicity
Chlorpromazine	Antacids	Complexes in gut lumen	Reduced chlorpromazine absorption
	Anticholinergics	Delayed gastric emptying	Reduced chlorpromazine bioavailablity
	Bethanidine	Inhibition of neuronal uptake	Reduced hypotension
	Debrisoquine	Inhibition of neuronal uptake	Reduced hypotension
	Guanethidine	Inhibition of neuronal uptake	Reduced hypotension
	Pethidine	Increased pethidine metabolites	Lethargy
	Phenytoin	Enzyme inhibition	Phenytoin toxicity
	Propranolol	Mutual enzyme inhibition	Potentiation of both
Chlorpropamide	Ethanol	Unknown	Facial flushing
	Phenylbutazone	Enzyme inhibition/ protein binding displacement	Hypoglycaemia
	Sulphonamides	Enzyme inhibition	Hypoglycaemia
Cholestyramine	Digitoxin	Binding in gut lumen	Reduced digitoxin effect
	Digoxin	Binding in gut lumen	Reduced digoxin effect
	Thyroxine	Binding in gut lumen	Reduced thyroxine effect
	Warfarin	Binding in gut lumen	Reduced anticoagulation

	Interacting drug	Mechanism	Possible outcome
Cimetidine	Carbamazepine	Enzyme inhibition	Carbamazepine toxicity
	Chlordiazepoxide	Enzyme inhibition	Increased circulating chlordiazepoxide
	Chlormethiazole	Enzyme inhibition	Chlormethiazole toxicity
	Clobazam	Enzyme inhibition	Increased circulating clobazam
	Diazepam	Enzyme inhibition	Increased circulating diazepam
	Imipramine	Enzyme inhibition	Imipramine toxicity
	Ketoconazole	Impaired absorption	Loss of ketoconazole effect
	Labetolol	Enzyme inhibition	Increased labetolol effect
	Lignocaine	Enzyme inhibition	Lignocaine toxicity
	Metoprolol	Enzyme inhibition	Increased metoprolol effect
	Nitrazepam	Enzyme inhibition	Increased circulating nitrazepam
	Phenytoin	Enzyme inhibition	Phenytoin toxicity
	Procainamide	Reduced renal excretion	Increased procainamide concentration
	Propranolol	Enzyme inhibition	Increased propranolol effect
	Quinidine	Enzyme inhibition	Quinidine toxicity
	Theophylline	Enzyme inhibition	Theophylline toxicity
	Triazolam	Enzyme inhibition	Increased circulating triazolam
	Warfarin	Enzyme inhibition	Potentiated anti-coagulation
Clindamycin	Neuromuscular blockers	Additive	Increased blockade
Clobazam	Cimetidine	Enzyme inhibition	Increased circulating clobazam
Clofibrate	Tolbutamide	Enzyme inhibition	Hypoglycaemia
	Warfarin	Uncertain	Potentiated anti-coagulation
Clonazepam	Carbamazepine	Enzyme induction	Reduced clonazepam concentration
Clonidine	Ethanol	Synergism	Sedation
	Tricyclic anti-depressants	Alpha receptor competition	Reduced hypotension
Colestipol	Digoxin	Binding in gut lumen	Reduced digoxin effect
Cyclophos-phamide	Allopurinol	Uncertain	Bone marrow toxicity
Cyclosporin	Ketoconazole	Enzyme inhibition	Cyclosporin nephro-toxicity
	Rifampicin	Enzyme induction	Transplant rejection

6

Drug Interactions

	Interacting drug	Mechanism	Possible outcome
Cytotoxic agents	Phenytoin	Reduced absorption	Breakthrough seizures
Danazol	Warfarin	Synergism	Potentiated anti-coagulation
Debrisoquine	Chlorpromazine	Inhibition of neuronal uptake	Reduced hypotension
	Ephedrine	Competition for neuronal uptake	Reduced hypotension
	Mazindol	Inhibition of neuronal uptake	Reduced hypotension
	Phenylephrine	Competition for neuronal uptake	Reduced hypotension
	Phenylpropanolamine	Competition for neuronal uptake	Reduced hypotension
	Pizotifen	Inhibition of neuronal uptake	Reduced hypotension
	Tricyclic anti-depressants	Inhibition of neuronal uptake	Reduced hypotension
Dexamethasone	Aminoglutethimide	Enzyme induction	Reduced steroid effect
	Phenytoin	Enzyme induction	Reduced steroid effect
Dextropropoxy-phene	Carbamazepine	Enzyme inhibition	Carbamazepine toxicity
	Doxepin	Enzyme inhibition	Increased circulating doxepin
	Phenobarbitone	Enzyme inhibition	Phenobarbitone toxicity
Diazepam	Cimetidine	Enzyme inhibition	Increased circulating diazepam
	Disulfiram	Enzyme inhibition	Increased circulating diazepam
	Ethanol	Synergism	Sedation
	Oral contraceptives	Enzyme inhibition	Increased circulating diazepam
	Phenytoin	Enzyme induction	Reduced diazepam effect
	Sodium valproate	Enzyme inhibition/ protein binding displacement	Increased diazepam effect
	Theophylline	Receptor antagonism	Reduced diazepam effect
Dichloral-phenazone	Warfarin	Enzyme induction	Reduced anti-coagulation
Diclofenac	Lithium	Reduction in renal excretion	Lithium toxicity
Digitoxin	Cholestyramine	Binding in gut lumen	Reduced digitoxin effect
	Phenobarbitone	Enzyme induction	Reduced digitoxin effect
	Rifampicin	Enzyme induction	Reduced digitoxin effect

	Interacting drug	Mechanism	Possible outcome
Digoxin	Amiodarone	Reduction in renal excretion	Digoxin toxicity
	Amphotericin	Production of hypo-kalaemia	Digoxin toxicity
	Antacids	Binding in gut lumen	Reduced digoxin effect
	Anticholinergics	Delayed gastric emptying	Increased digoxin absorption
	Bumetanide	Production of hypo-kalaemia	Digoxin toxicity
	Cholestyramine	Binding in gut lumen	Reduced digoxin effect
	Colestipol	Binding in gut lumen	Reduced digoxin effect
	Erythromycin	Decreased gut metabolism	Increased digoxin bioavailability
	Frusemide	Production of hypo-kalaemia	Digoxin toxicity
	Kaolin-pectin mixtures	Binding in gut lumen	Reduced digoxin effect
	Neomycin	Impaired absorption	Reduced digoxin effect
	Quinidine	Reduction in renal excretion	Digoxin toxicity
	Quinine	Reduction in renal excretion	Digoxin toxicity
	Spironolactone	Inhibition of tubular secretion	Digoxin toxicity
	Tetracyclines	Decreased gut metabolism	Increased digoxin effect
	Thiazide diuretics	Production of hypo-kalaemia	Digoxin toxicity
	Verapamil	Reduction in renal excetion	Digoxin toxicity
Disopyramide	Amiodarone	Synergism	Ventricular arrhythmias
	Quinidine	Small increase in concentration	Possible quinidine toxicity
Disulfiram	Chlordiazepoxide	Enzyme inhibition	Increased circulating chlordiazepoxide
	Diazepam	Enzyme inhibition	Increased circulating diazepam
	Ethanol	Inhibition of acetal-dehyde oxidation	Antabuse reaction
	Phenytoin	Enzyme inhibition	Phenytoin toxicity
	Warfarin	Enzyme inhibition	Potentiated anti-coagulation
Doxepin	Dextropropoxy-phene	Enzyme inhibition	Increased circulating doxepin
Ephedrine	Bethanidine	Inhibition of neuronal uptake	Reduced hypotension
	Debrisoquine	Inhibition of neuronal uptake	Reduced hypotension
	Guanethidine	Inhibition of neuronal uptake	Reduced hypotension

6

Drug Interactions

	Interacting drug	Mechanism	Possible outcome
Erythromycin	Carbamazepine	Enzyme inhibition	Carbamazepine toxicity
	Digoxin	Decreased gut metabolism	Increased digoxin bioavailability
	Methylprednisolone	Enzyme inhibition	Increased steroid effect
	Theophylline	Enzyme inhibition	Theophylline toxicity
	Warfarin	Enzyme inhibition	Potentiated anti-coagulation
Ethacrynic acid	Aminoglycosides	Additive	Nephrotoxicity, ototoxicity
	Cephaloridine	Increased intra-renal concentration	Nephrotoxicity
Ethambutol	Antacids	Decreased absorption	Treatment failure
Ethanol	Chloral hydrate	Inhibition of acetal-dehyde oxidation	Antabuse reaction
	Chlordiazepoxide	Enzyme inhibition	Increased circulating chlordiazepoxide
	Chlorpropamide	Unknown	Facial flushing
	Clonidine	Synergism	Sedation
	Diazepam	Synergism	Sedation
	Disulfiram	Inhibition of acetal-dehyde oxidation	Antabuse reaction
	Insulin	Insulin release	Potentiation of hypoglycaemia
	Methyldopa	Additive	Sedation
	Metronidazole	Inhibition of acetal-dehyde oxidation	Antabuse reaction
	Nitrazepam	Additive	Sedation
	Phenformin	Synergism	Lactic acidosis
	Phenobarbitone	Synergism	Sedation
	Phenytoin	Enzyme induction	Reduced phenytoin effect
	Procarbazine	Inhibition of acetal-dehyde oxidation	Antabuse reaction
	Tolbutamide	Enzyme inhibition/induction	Hypoglycaemia/hyperglycaemia
	Tricyclic anti-depressants	Synergism	Psychomotor impairment
Ethosuximide	Carbamazepine	Enzyme induction	Decreased ethosuximide effect
	Sodium valproate	Enzyme inhibition	Increased ethosuximide effect
Flurbiprofen	Frusemide	Antagonism	Reduced diuresis
Frusemide	Aminoglycosides	Reduced renal excretion	Ototoxicity, nephro-toxicity
	Cephaloridine	Increased intra-renal concentration	Nephrotoxicity
	Digoxin	Production of hypo-kalaemia	Digoxin toxicity
	Flurbiprofen	Antagonism	Reduced diuresis
	Indomethacin	Antagonism	Reduced diuresis
	Lithium	Increased tubular re-absorption	Lithium toxicity

6

Drug Interactions

	Interacting drug	Mechanism	Possible outcome
Glutethimide	Warfarin	Enzyme induction	Reduced anti-coagulation
Glyceryl trinitrate	Phenobarbitone	Enzyme induction	Reduced nitrate effect
Griseofulvin	Oral contraceptives	Enzyme induction	Breakthrough bleeding
	Phenobarbitone	Enzyme induction	Reduced griseofulvin effect
	Warfarin	Enzyme induction	Reduced anticoagulation
Guanethidine	Chlorpromazine	Inhibition of neuronal uptake	Reduced hypotension
	Ephedrine	Competition for neuronal uptake	Reduced hypotension
	Haloperidol	Inhibition of neuronal uptake	Reduced hypotension
	Mazindol	Inhibition of neuronal uptake	Reduced hypotension
	Phenylephrine	Competition for neuronal uptake	Reduced hypotension
	Phenylpropanolamine	Competition for neuronal uptake	Reduced hypotension
	Pizotifen	Inhibition of neuronal uptake	Reduced hypotension
	Tricyclic anti-depressants	Inhibition of neuronal uptake	Reduced hypotension
Haloperidol	Guanethidine	Inhibition of neuronal uptake	Reduced hypotension
	Indomethacin	Unknown	Increased sedation
	Lithium	Synergism	Neurotoxicity
	Methyldopa	Synergism	Sedation, aggression
Hydrocortisone	Phenobarbitone	Enzyme induction	Loss of steroid effect
	Phenytoin	Enzyme induction	Loss of steroid effect
	Rifampicin	Enzyme induction	Addisonian crisis
Imipramine	Cimetidine	Enzyme inhibition	Imipramine toxicity
	Phenytoin	Enzyme inhibition	Phenytoin toxicity
Indomethacin	Bumetanide	Antagonism	Reduced diuresis
	Captopril	Unknown	Reduction in captopril effect
	Frusemide	Antagonism	Reduced diuresis
	Haloperidol	Unknown	Increased sedation
	Lithium	Reduction in renal excretion	Lithium toxicity
	Oxprenolol	Inhibition of renal prostaglandin synthesis	Reduced hypotension
	Probenecid	Inhibition of tubular secretion	Increased circulating indomethacin
	Propranolol	Inhibition of renal prostaglandin synthesis	Reduced hypotension
	Thiazide diuretics	Inhibition of renal prostaglandin synthesis	Reduced hypotension

6

Drug Interactions

	Interacting drug	Mechanism	Possible outcome
Insulin	Atenolol	Blocking cardiovascular response	Masking hypoglycaemic symptoms
	Ethanol	Insulin release	Potentiation of hypo-glycaemia
	Metoprolol	Blocking cardiovascular response	Masking hypoglycaemic symptoms
	Monoamine oxidase inhibitors	Insulin release/ blocking adrenergic responses	Hypoglycaemia
	Oxprenolol	Interference with glycogenolysis/ blocking cardio-vascular response	Prolongation of hypo-glycaemia/masking hypoglycaemic symptoms
	Propranolol	Interference with glycogenolysis/ blocking cardio-vascular response	Prolongation of hypo-glycaemia/masking hypoglycaemic symptoms
Iodides	Lithium	Reduced thyroid hormone synthesis and release	Hypothyroidism
Iron	Antacids	Insoluble complexes in gut lumen	Reduced iron absorption
	Penicillamine	Complexes in gut lumen	Reduced penicillamine effect
	Tetracyclines	Insoluble complexes in gut lumen	Treatment failure
Isoniazid	Antacids	Decreased absorption	Treatment failure
	Carbamazepine	Enzyme inhibition	Carbamazepine toxicity
	Phenytoin	Enzyme inhibition	Phenytoin toxicity
	Triazolam	Enzyme inhibition	Increased circulating triazolam
	Warfarin	Enzyme inhibition	Potentiated anti-coagulation
Kaolin-pectin mixtures	Digoxin	Binding in gut lumen	Reduced digoxin effect
	Lincomycin	Binding in gut lumen	Treatment failure
Ketoconazole	Antacids	Impaired absorption	Loss of ketaconazole effect
	Cyclosporin	Enzyme inhibition	Cyclosporin nephrotoxicity
	Cimetidine	Impaired absorption	Loss of ketoconazole effect
	Ranitidine	Impaired absorption	Loss of ketoconazole effect
	Warfarin	Enzyme inhibition	Potentiated anti-coagulation
Labetalol	Cimetidine	Enzyme inhibition	Increased labetolol effect

Drug Interactions

6

	Interacting drug	Mechanism	Possible outcome
Levodopa	Antacids	Increased gastric emptying	Enhanced levodopa absorption
	Metoclopramide	Increased gastric emptying	Enhanced levodopa effect
	Monoamine oxidase inhibitors	Increased intrasynaptic dompamine	Hypertension
	Tricyclic anti-depressants	Inhibition of dopamine uptake	Sympathetic over-activity
Lignocaine	Cimetidine	Enzyme inhibition	Lignocaine toxicity
	Propranolol	Reduction in clearance	Lignocaine toxicity
Lincomycin	Kaolin-pectin mixtures	Binding in gut lumen	Treatment failure
Lithium	Acetazolamide	Increased renal excretion	Reduced lithium effect
	Anticholinergics	Delayed gastric emptying	Reduced lithium absorption
	Bumetanide	Increased tubular reabsorption	Lithium toxicity
	Carbamazepine	Synergism	Lithium toxicity
	Diclofenac	Reduction in renal excretion	Lithium toxicity
	Frusemide	Increased tubular reabsorption	Lithium toxicity
	Haloperidol	Synergism	Neurotoxicity
	Indomethacin	Reduction in renal excretion	Lithium toxicity
	Iodides	Reduced thyroid hormone synthesis and release	Hypothyroidism
	Mazindol	Unclear	Lithium toxicity
	Neuroleptics	Synergism	Neurotoxicity
	Neuromuscular blockers	Impedance of pre-synaptic transmission	Increased blockade
	Phenylbutazone	Reduction in renal excretion	Lithium toxicity
	Phenytoin	Synergism	Lithium toxicity
	Piroxicam	Reduction in renal excretion	Lithium toxicity
	Tetracycline	Renal tubular damage	Lithium toxicity
	Thiazide diuretics	Increased tubular reabsorption	Lithium toxicity
Mazindol	Bethanidine	Inhibition of neuronal uptake	Reduced hypotension
	Debrisoquine	Inhibition of neuronal uptake	Reduced hypotension
	Guanethidine	Inhibition of neuronal uptake	Reduced hypotension
	Lithium	Unclear	Lithium toxicity
Mercaptopurine	Allopurinol	Enzyme inhibition	Mercaptopurine toxicity
Methadone	Rifampicin	Enzyme induction	Withdrawal syndrome

	Interacting drug	Mechanism	Possible outcome
Methotrexate	Aspirin	Competition for active renal transport	Methotrexate toxicity
	Phenylbutazone	Competition for active renal transport	Methotrexate toxicity
	Probenecid	Competition for active renal transport	Methotrexate toxicity
	Sulphonamides	Protein-binding displacement	Methotrexate toxicity
Methyldopa	Ethanol	Additive	Sedation
	Haloperidol	Synergism	Sedation, aggression
	Monoamine oxidase inhibitors	Unclear	Excitement, sweating, rigidity
	Tricyclic anti-depressants	Inhibition of amine uptake	Reduced hypotensive effect
Methyl-prednisolone	Erythromycin	Enzyme inhibition	Increased steroid effect
	Phenytoin	Enzyme induction	Loss of steroid effect
	Rifampicin	Enzyme induction	Loss of transplant function
Metoclopramide	Levodopa	Increased gastric emptying	Enhanced levodopa effect
Metoprolol	Cimetidine	Enzyme inhibition	Increased metoprolol effect
	Insulin	Blocking cardio-vascular resonse	Masking hypoglycaemic symptoms
Metronidazole	Ethanol	Inhibition of acetal-dehyde oxidation	Antabuse reaction
	Phenytoin	Enzyme inhibition	Phenytoin toxicity
	Warfarin	Enzyme inhibition	Potentiated anti-coagulation
Mexilitine	Acetazolamide	Decreased excretion	Increased circulating mexilitine
	Phenytoin	Enzyme induction	Reduced mexilitine effect
Miconazole	Phenytoin	Enzyme inhibition	Phenytoin toxicity
Monoamine oxidase inhibitors	Amphetamines	Increased intra-synaptic amines	Severe hypertension
	Insulin	Insulin release/ blocking adrenergic responses	Hypoglycaemia
	Levodopa	Increased intra-synaptic dopamine	Hypertension
	Methyldopa	Unclear	Excitement, sweating, rigidity
	Pethidine	Unclear	Excitement, sweating, rigidity, hypertension
	Phenylpropanolamine	Indirect sympatho-mimetic effect	Severe sympathetic overactivity with hypertension

	Interacting drug	Mechanism	Possible outcome
Monoamine oxidase inhibitors (Contd.)	Pseudoephedrine	Indirect sympatho-mimetic effect	Severe sympathetic overactivity with hypertension
	Reserpine	Noradrenaline release	CNS excitation
	Tricyclic anti-depressants	Synergism	Sympathetic overactivity
	Tyramine containing foods	Indirect sympatho-mimetic effect	Severe sympathetic overactivity with hypertension
Neomycin	Digoxin	Impaired absorption	Reduced digoxin effect
	Oral contraceptives	Interference with steroid hydrolysis	Contraceptive failure
Neuroleptics	Lithium	Synergism	Neurotoxicity
	Tricyclic anti-depressants	Mutual enzyme inhibition	Potentiation of both
Neuromuscular blockers	Aminoglycosides	Additive	Increased blockade
	Amphotericin	Production of hypo-kalaemia	Potentiation
	Clindamycin	Additive	Increased blockade
	Lithium	Impedence of pre-synaptic transmission	Increased blockade
	Quinidine	Additive	Increased blockade
Nifedipine	Propranolol	Synergistic cardio-depression	Cardiac failure
Nitrazepam	Cimetidine	Enzyme inhibition	Increased circulating nitrazepam
	Ethanol	Additive	Sedation
Oral contraceptives	Ampicillin	Reduced enterohepatic circulation	Contraceptive failure
	Broad spectrum antibiotics	Reduced enterohepatic circulation	Contraceptive failure
	Carbamazepine	Enzyme induction	Contraceptive failure
	Chlordiazepoxide	Enzyme inhibition	Increased circulating chlordiazepoxide
	Diazepam	Enzyme inhibition	Increased circulating diazepam
	Griseofulvin	Enzyme induction	Breakthrough bleeding
	Neomycin	Interference with steroid hydrolysis	Contraceptive failure
	Phenobarbitone	Enzyme induction	Contraceptive failure
	Phenytoin	Enzyme induction	Contraceptive failure
	Prednisolone	Enzyme inhibition	Increased steroid effect
	Primidone	Enzyme induction	Contraceptive failure
	Rifampicin	Enzyme induction	Contraceptive failure
	Tetracyclines	Reduced enterohepatic circulation	Contraceptive failure
	Theophylline	Enzyme inhibition	Increased circulating theophylline

6

Drug Interactions

	Interacting drug	Mechanism	Possible outcome
Oxprenolol	Indomethacin	Inhibition of renal prostaglandin synthesis	Reduced hypotension
	Insulin	Interference with glycogenolysis/ blocking cardio-vascular response	Prolongation of hypo-glycaemia/masking hypoglycaemic symptoms
Oxyphenbutazone	Tolbutamide	Enzyme inhibition	Hypoglycaemia
	Warfarin	Enzyme inhibition	Potentiated anticoagulation
Penicillamine	Antacids	Binding in gut lumen	Reduced penicillamine absorption
	Iron	Complexes in gut lumen	Reduced penicillamine effect
Penicillins	Aminoglycosides	Incompatibility in infusions	Treatment failure
	Probenecid	Competition for active renal transport	Increased circulating penicillin
Pethidine	Chlorpromazine	Increased pethidine metabolites	Lethargy
	Monoamine oxidase inhibitors	Unknown	Excitement, sweating, rigidity, hypertension
	Phenytoin	Enzyme induction	Reduced analgesia
Phenformin	Ethanol	Synergism	Lactic acidosis
	Tetracyclines	Unknown	Lactic acidosis
Phenobarbitone	Dextropropoxyphene	Enzyme inhibition	Phenobarbitone toxicity
	Digitoxin	Enzyme induction	Reduced digitoxin effect
	Ethanol	Synergism	Sedation
	Glyceryl trinitrate	Enzyme induction	Reduced nitrate effect
	Griseofulvin	Enzyme induction	Reduced griseofulvin effect
	Hydrocortisone	Enzyme inducton	Loss of steroid effect
	Oral contraceptives	Enzyme induction	Contraceptive failure
	Rifampicin	Enzyme induction	Increase in seizure frequency
	Sodium valproate	Enzyme inhibition	Increased phenobarbitone effect
	Testosterone	Enzyme induction	Reduced steroid effect
	Tricyclic anti-depressants	Enzyme induction	Breakthrough depression
	Warfarin	Enzyme induction	Reduced anticoagulation
Phenylbutazone	Acetohexamide	Reduced excretion of active metabolites	Hypoglycaemia
	Chlorpropamide	Enzyme inhibition/ protein binding displacement	Hypoglycaemia

	Interacting drug	Mechanism	Possible outcome
Phenylbutazone (Contd.)	Lithium	Reduction in renal excretion	Lithium toxicity
	Methotrexate	Competition for active renal transport	Methotrexate toxicity
	Phenytoin	Enzyme inhibition/ protein binding displacement	Phenytoin toxicity
	Tolbutamide	Enzyme inhibition	Hypoglycaemia
	Warfarin	Enzyme inhibition/ protein binding displacement	Potentiated anti-coagulation
Phenylephrine	Bethanidine	Competition for neuronal uptake	Reduced hypotension
	Debrisoquine	Competition for neuronal uptake	Reduced hypotension
	Guanethidine	Competition for neuronal uptake	Reduced hypotension
Phenylpropanol-amine	Bethanidine	Competition for neuronal uptake	Reduced hypotension
	Debrisoquine	Competition for neuronal uptake	Reduced hypotension
	Guanethidine	Competition for neuronal uptake	Reduced hypotension
	Monoamine oxidase inhibitors	Indirect sympatho-mimetic effect	Severe sympathetic overactivity with hypertension
Phenytoin	Allopurinol	Enzyme inhibition	Phenytoin toxicity
	Azapropazone	Enzyme inhibition	Phenytoin toxicity
	Carbamazepine	Mutual enzyme induction	Reduced concentration of both
	Chloramphenicol	Enzyme inhibition	Phenytoin toxicity
	Chlorpromazine	Enzyme inhibition	Phenytoin toxicity
	Cimetidine	Enzyme inhibition	Phenytoin toxicity
	Cytotoxic agents	Reduced absorption	Breakthrough seizures
	Dexamethasone	Enzyme induction	Reduced steroid effect
	Diazepam	Enzyme induction	Reduced diazepam effect
	Disulfiram	Enzyme inhibition	Phenytoin toxicity
	Ethanol	Enzyme induction	Reduced phenytoin effect
	Hydrocortisone	Enzyme inducton	Reduced steroid effect
	Imipramine	Enzyme inhibition	Phenytoin toxicity
	Isoniazid	Enzyme inhibition	Phenytoin toxicity
	Lithium	Synergism	Lithium toxicity
	Methylprednisolone	Enzyme induction	Loss of steroid effect
	Metronidazole	Enzyme inhibition	Phenytoin toxicity
	Mexilitine	Enzyme induction	Reduced mexilitine effect
	Miconazole	Enzyme inhibition	Phenytoin toxicity
	Oral contraceptives	Enzyme induction	Contraceptive failure
	Pethidine	Enzyme induction	Reduced analgesia
	Phenylbutazone	Enzyme inhibition/ protein binding displacement	Phenytoin toxicity
	Prednisolone	Enzyme induction	Loss of steroid effect
	Quinidine	Enzyme induction	Breakthrough arrhythmia

6

Drug Interactions

	Interacting drug	Mechanism	Possible outcome
Phenytoin (Contd.)	Sodium valproate	Enzyme induction	Reduced valproate concentration
		Enzyme inhibition/ protein binding displacement	Phenytoin toxicity
	Sulphonamides	Enzyme inhibition	Phenytoin toxicity
	Sulthiame	Enzyme inhibition	Phenytoin toxicity
	Thioridazine	Enzyme inhibition	Phenytoin toxicity
	Thyroxine	Enzyme induction	Reduced thyroxine effect
	Warfarin	Enzyme induction	Reduced anticoagulation
Piroxicam	Lithium	Reduction in renal excretion	Lithium toxicity
Pizotifen	Bethanidine	Inhibition of neuronal uptake	Reduced hypotension
	Debrisoquine	Inhibition of neuronal uptake	Reduced hypotension
	Guanethidine	Inhibition of neuronal uptake	Reduced hypotension
Polymixins	Aminoglycosides	Additive	Nephrotoxicity
	Neuromuscular blockers	Additive	Increased blockade
Potassium supplements	Amiloride	Additive	Hyperkalaemia
	Captopril	Additive	Hyperkalaemia
	Spironolactone	Additive	Hyperkalaemia
	Triamterene	Additive	Hyperkalaemia
Prednisolone	Oral contraceptives	Enzyme inhibition	Increased steroid effect
	Phenytoin	Enzyme induction	Loss of steroid effect
	Rifampicin	Enzyme induction	Loss of steroid effect
Primidone	Oral contraceptives	Enzyme induction	Contraceptive failure
Probenecid	Aspirin	Antagonism	Loss of uricosuric effect
	Cephalosporins	Competition for active renal transport	Increased circulating cephalosporin
	Indomethacin	Inhibition of tubular secretion	Increased circulating indomethacin
	Methotrexate	Competition for active renal transport	Methotrexate toxicity
	Penicillins	Competition for active renal transport	Increased circulating penicillin
Procainamide	Cimetidine	Reduced renal excretion	Increased procainamide concentration
Procarbazine	Ethanol	Inhibition of acetal- dehyde oxidation	Antabuse reaction

	Interacting drug	Mechanism	Possible outcome
Propranolol	Chlorpromazine	Mutual enzyme inhibition	Potentiation of both
	Cimetidine	Enzyme inhibition	Increased propranolol effect
	Indomethacin	Inhibition of renal prostaglandin synthesis	Reduced hypotension
	Insulin	Interference with glycogenolysis/ blocking cardio- vascular response	Prolongation of hypo- glycaemia/masking hypoglycaemic symptoms
	Lignocaine	Reduction in clearance	Lignocaine toxicity
	Nifedipine	Synergistic cardio- depression	Cardiac failure
	Theophylline	Enzyme inhibition	Theophylline toxicity
	Verapamil	Synergism	Cardiac failure, con- duction defects
Pseudoephedrine	Monoamine oxidase inhibitors	Indirect sympatho- mimetic effect	Severe sympathetic overactivity with hypertension
Quinidine	Acetazolamide	Decreased excretion	Increased circulating quinidine
	Amiodarone	Enzyme inhibition	Quinidine toxicity
	Antacids	Reduced tubular reabsorption	Increased renal quinidine excretion
	Cimetidine	Enzyme inhibition	Quinidine toxicity
	Digoxin	Reduction in renal excretion	Digoxin toxicity
	Disopyramide	Small increase in concentration	Possible quinidine toxicity
	Neuromuscular blockers	Additive	Increased blockade
	Phenytoin	Enzyme induction	Breakthrough arrhythmia
	Rifampicin	Enzyme induction	Recurrence of arrhythmia
	Warfarin	Uncertain	Potentiated anti- coagulation
Quinine	Digoxin	Reduction in renal excretion	Digoxin toxicity
Ranitidine	Ketoconazole	Impaired absorption	Loss of ketoconazole effect
Reserpine	Monoamine oxidase inhibitors	Noradrenaline release	CNS excitation
Rifampicin	Cyclosporin	Enzyme induction	Transplant rejection
	Digitoxin	Enzyme induction	Reduced digitoxin effect
	Hydrocortisone	Enzyme induction	Addisonian crisis
	Methadone	Enzyme induction	Withdrawal syndrome
	Methylprednisolone	Enzyme induction	Loss of transplant function
	Oral contraceptives	Enzyme induction	Contraceptive failure
	Phenobarbitone	Enzyme induction	Increase in seizure frequency

	Interacting drug	Mechanism	Possible outcome
Rifampicin (Contd.)	Prednisolone	Enzyme induction	Loss of steroid effect
	Quinidine	Enzyme induction	Recurrence of arrhythmia
	Tolbutamide	Enzyme induction	Hyperglycaemia
	Warfarin	Enzyme induction	Reduced anti-coagulation
Sodium valproate	Carbamazepine	Enzyme induction	Reduced valproate concentration
	Diazepam	Enzyme inhibition/ protein binding displacement	Increased diazepam effect
	Ethosuximide	Enzyme inhibition	Increased ethosuximide effect
	Phenobarbitone	Enzyme inhibition	Increased phenobarbitone effect
	Phenytoin	Enzyme induction	Reduced valproate concentration
		Enzyme inhibition/ protein binding displacement	Phenytoin toxicity
Spironolactone	Carbenoxolone	Antagonism	Inhibition of ulcer healing
	Digoxin	Inhibition of tubular secretion	Digoxin toxicity
	Potassium supplements	Additive	Hyperkalaemia
Sucralfate	Warfarin	Binding in gut lumen	Reduced anti-coagulation
Sulphinpyrazone	Phenytoin	Enzyme inhibition	Phenytoin toxicity
	Theophylline	Enzyme induction	Reduced theophylline effect
	Tolbutamide	Enzyme inhibition	Hypoglycaemia
	Warfarin	Enzyme inhibition	Potentiated anti-coagulation
Sulphonamides	Methotrexate	Protein binding displacement	Methotrexate toxicity
	Phenytoin	Enzyme inhibition	Phenytoin toxicity
	Tolbutamide	Enzyme inhibition	Hypoglycaemia
	Warfarin	Enzyme inhibition	Potentiated anti-coagulation
Sulthiame	Phenytoin	Enzyme inhibition	Phenytoin toxicity
Testosterone	Phenobarbitone	Enzyme induction	Reduced steroid effect
Tetracyclines	Antacids	Insoluble complexes in gut lumen	Treatment failure
	Digoxin	Decreased gut metabolism	Increased digoxin effect
	Iron	Insoluble complexes in gut lumen	Treatment failure
	Lithium	Renal tubular damage	Lithium toxicity

	Interacting drug	Mechanism	Possible outcome
Tetracyclines (Contd.)	Oral contraceptives	Reduced enterohepatic circulation	Contraceptive failure
	Phenformin	Unknown	Lactic acidosis
Theophylline	Allopurinol	Enzyme inhibition	Theophylline toxicity
	Carbamazepine	Enzyme induction	Reduced theophylline effect
	Cimetidine	Enzyme inhibition	Theophylline toxicity
	Diazepam	Receptor antagonism	Reduced diazepam effect
	Erythromycin	Enzyme inhibition	Theophylline toxicity
	Oral contraceptives	Enzyme inhibition	Increased circulating theophylline
	Propranolol	Enzyme inhibition	Theophylline toxicity
	Sulphinpyrazone	Enzyme induction	Reduced theophylline effect
Thiazide diuretics	Digoxin	Production of hypo-kalaemia	Digoxin toxicity
	Indomethacin	Inhibition of renal prostaglandin synthesis	Reduced hypotension
	Lithium	Increased tubular reabsorption	Lithium toxicity
Thioridazine	Phenytoin	Enzyme inhibition	Phenytoin toxicity
Thyroxine	Cholestyramine	Binding in gut lumen	Reduced thyroxine effect
	Phenytoin	Enzyme induction	Reduced thyroxine effect
Tolbutamide	Azapropazone	Enzyme inhibition	Hypoglycaemia
	Chloramphenicol	Enzyme inhibition	Hypoglycaemia
	Clofibrate	Enzyme inhibition	Hypoglycaemia
	Ethanol (acute)	Enzyme inhibition	Hypoglycaemia
	Ethanol (chronic)	Enzyme induction	Hyperglycaemia
	Oxyphenbutazone	Enzyme inhibition	Hypoglycaemia
	Phenylbutazone	Enzyme inhibition	Hypoglycaemia
	Rifampicin	Enzyme induction	Hyperglycaemia
	Sulphinpyrazone	Enzyme inhibition	Hypoglycaemia
	Sulphonamides	Enzyme inhibition	Hypoglycaemia
Triamterene	Potassium supplements	Additive	Hyperkalaemia
Triazolam	Cimetidine	Enzyme inhibition	Increased circulating triazolam
	Isoniazid	Enzyme inhibition	Increased circulating triazolam
Tricyclic anti-depressants	Anticholinergics	Synergism	Anticholinergic side effects
	Bethanidine	Inhibition of neuronal uptake	Reduced hypotension
	Clonidine	Alpha receptor competition	Reduced hypotension
	Debrisoquine	Inhibition of neuronal uptake	Reduced hypotension

6

Drug interactions

	Interacting drug	Mechanism	Possible outcome
Tricyclic anti-depressants (Contd.)	Ethanol	Synergism	Psychomotor impairment
	Guanethidine	Inhibition of neuronal uptake	Reduced hypotension
	Levodopa	Inhibition of dopamine uptake	Sympathetic overactivity
	Methyldopa	Inhibition of amine uptake	Reduced hypotensive effect
	Monoamine oxidase inhibitors	Synergism	Sympathetic overactivity
	Neuroleptics	Mutual enzyme inhibition	Potentiation of both
	Phenobarbitone	Enzyme induction	Breakthrough depression
Tyramine-containing foods (e.g. cheese, tomatoes, chocolate bananas, yeast products, red wine, pickled herring, meat extracts)	Monoamine oxidase inhibitors	Indirect sympatho-mimetic effect	Severe sympathetic overactivity with hypertension
Verapamil	Atenolol	Synergism	Cardiac failure, conduction defects
	Digoxin	Reduction in renal excretion	Digoxin toxicity
	Propanolol	Synergism	Cardiac failure, conduction defects
Warfarin	Allopurinol	Enzyme inhibition	Potentiated anticoagulation
	Aminoglutethimide	Enzyme induction	Reduced anticoagulation
	Amiodarone	Enzyme inhibition	Potentiated anticoagulation
	Anabolic steroids	Synergism	Potentiated anticoagulation
	Aspirin	Synergism	Haemorrhage
	Azapropazone	Enzyme inhibition	Potentiated anticoagulation
	Carbamazepine	Enzyme induction	Reduced anticoagulation
	Chloramphenicol	Enzyme inhibition	Potentiated anticoagulation
	Cholestyramine	Binding in gut lumen	Reduced anticoagulation
	Cimetidine	Enzyme inhibition	Potentiated anticoagulation
	Clofibrate	Uncertain	Potentiated anticoagulation
	Danazol	Synergism	Potentiated anticoagulation
	Dichloralphenazone	Enzyme induction	Reduced anticoagulation
	Disulfiram	Enzyme inhibition	Potentiated anticoagulation

6

Drug Interactions

	Interacting drug	Mechanism	Possible outcome
Warfarin (Contd.)	Erythromycin	Enzyme inhibition	Potentiated anticoagulation
	Ethanol	Enzyme induction	Reduced anticoagulation
	Glutethimide	Enzyme induction	Reduced anticoagulation
	Griseofulvin	Enzyme induction	Reduced anticoagulation
	Isoniazid	Enzyme inhibition	Potentiated anticoagulation
	Ketoconazole	Enzyme inhibition	Potentiated anticoagulation
	Metronidazole	Enzyme inhibition	Potentiated anticoagulation
	Oxyphenbutazone	Enzyme inhibition	Potentiated anticoagulation
	Phenobarbitone	Enzyme induction	Reduced anticoagulation
	Phenylbutazone	Enzyme inhibition/ protein binding displacement	Potentiated anticoagulation
	Phenytoin	Enzyme induction	Reduced anticoagulation
	Quinidine	Uncertain	Potentiated anticoagulation
	Rifampicin	Enzyme induction	Reduced anticoagulation
	Sucralfate	Binding in gut lumen	Reduced anticoagulation
	Sulphinpyrazone	Enzyme inhibition	Potentiated anticoagulation
	Sulphonamides	Enzyme inhibition	Potentiated anticoagulation

6

Drug Interactions

7

Cautions

PRESCRIBING CAVEATS

There are a number of preparations available which have a poor risk/benefit ratio and cannot now be recommended. In some instances these are superseded drugs (e.g. reserpine), formulations (e.g. sustained release iron) or combinations (e.g. compound bronchodilator preparations). In others they are more expensive than existing preparations with no obvious increase in benefit, e.g. expensive diuretics, ampicillin esters. Some have not been shown to be clinically effective, e.g. mucolytics, cerebral vasodilators and others have greater toxicity than rival preparations, e.g. neomycin eye and ear preparations. Some drugs should be avoided for particular indications (e.g. long half-life benzodiazepines as hypnotics) or in particular patient groups (e.g. chlorpropamide in the elderly) or disease states (e.g. antidiarrhoeal drugs in bowel infections).

Preparation	Caveat
ADRENERGIC NEURONE BLOCKERS e.g. guanethidine, bethanidine, debrisoquine	Postural hypotension Sexual difficulties Largely superseded
AMPICILLIN ESTERS e.g. bacampicillin, pivampicillin talampicillin	Hydrolysed to ampicillin Expensive
ANTIDIARRHOEALS e.g. Lomotil, loperamide	Avoid in infective diarrhoea Delays eradication of organism
APPETITE SUPPRESSANTS (centrally acting) e.g. diethylpropion, fenfluramine mazindol, phentermine	Limited efficacy CNS side-effects Risk of dependence
BARBITURATE SEDATIVES e.g. amylobarbitone, butobarbitone, cyclobarbitone, pentobarbitone	Cerebral depressants Risk of dependence Fatal in overdose
BELLADONNA ALKALOIDS e.g. Neutradonna, Peptard	Anticholinergic side-effects Superseded by more selective agents
BENZODIAZEPINES (LONG HALF-LIFE) e.g. diazepam, nitrazepam, flurazepam	Avoid as hypnotics Hangover effects
BETA AGONISTS (NON-SELECTIVE) e.g. isoprenaline, orciprenaline	Risk of arrhythmias Use β_2 agonist
BRONCHODILATORS (COMPOUND PREPARATIONS) e.g. Amesec, Brovon, Asmapax, Medihaler-duo, Tedral	Potential toxicity Superseded
BRONCHODILATOR/SEDATIVE COMBINATIONS e.g. Expansyl, Franol, Phyldrox	Respiratory depression Superseded

Preparation	Caveat
CEREBRAL VASODILATORS e.g. co-dergocrine, cyclandelate, isoxsuprine, naftidrofuryl	Little evidence of vasodilator effect on diseased vessels
CHLORPROPAMIDE	Long half-life Avoid in elderly
CLINDAMYCIN	Risk of pseudomembranous colitis
CLOFIBRATE	Benefit outweighed by long-term adverse effects e.g. gallstones, malignancy
CLONIDINE	Sedation Anticholinergic effects Rebound hypertension on withdrawal
CO-TRIMOXAZOLE	Too toxic for minor infections such as urinary tract infections
COUGH SUPPRESSANT/EXPECTORANT COMBINATIONS e.g. Benylin	Ineffective for productive coughs Sedative
CYANOCOBALAMIN	Replaced by hydroxycobalamin which has longer duration of effect
DEXTROPROPOXYPHENE	Equivalent analgesia to aspirin and paracetamol Risk of dependence and fatal overdose
DIURETIC/POTASSIUM COMBINATIONS e.g. Navidrex K, Hydrosaluric K, Lasical, Burinex K, Neonaclex K	Insufficient potassium More expensive than diuretic alone
DIURETICS (NEW) e.g. clopamide, indapamide, mefruside, metolazone, xipamide	No therapeutic advantage over thiazides and much more expensive
ETHACRYNIC ACID	More toxic than frusemide and bumetanide
IRON (SUSTAINED RELEASE) e.g. Feospan	Poor bioavailability Expensive
LEVODOPA (alone)	Use with dopa decarboxylase inhibitor (Madopar or Sinemet)
LINCOMYCIN	Risk of pseudomembranous colitis
METHYSERGIDE	Rarely retroperitoneal fibrosis Seldom required
MUCOLYTICS e.g. acetylcysteine, carbocisteine, bromhexine, methylcysteine	Little evidence of clinical benefit
NEOMYCIN-CONTAINING EAR AND EYE PREPARATIONS	Local sensitisation rash similar clinically to original condition

7

Cautions

Preparation	Caveat
PHENOBARBITONE (in adults)	Sedative; withdrawal seizures Avoid as monotherapy
POTASSIUM SUPPLEMENTS e.g. Slow K, Sando-K, Kloref, Kay-Cee-L	Gastrointestinal irritation, bleeding or perforation can occur Should not be used routinely Potassium-sparing diuretic more pharmacologically precise
PRIMIDONE (in adults)	Sedative; withdrawal seizures Avoid as monotherapy
RESERPINE	Central side-effects e.g. depression Superseded
SULTHIAME	Toxic Low efficacy
XANTHINE COUGH SYRUPS e.g. Franolyn, Nethaprin	Ineffective Potentially toxic if recommended dose is exceeded

7

Cautions

PAEDIATRIC PRESCRIBING

Little is known about the differences in drug handling and response in children in comparison with adults. Hepatic metabolism is slow in the premature infant but faster in the neonate and toddler than in the adult, as the liver volume per unit body weight decreases with age throughout childhood. During the first year of life renal excretion mechanisms reach adult capacity. The pharmacological response to a drug in children may differ from that in the adult, e.g. cerebral stimulation with phenobarbitone, greater tolerance to digoxin. A particularly selective policy of prescribing for children is advised. As in the adult, clinical monitoring of response should be attempted whenever possible. There are two methods of calculating paediatric doses. In pre-school children a mg/kg body weight is usually used, for example:

$$\frac{\text{Adult dose (mg)}}{70 \text{ kg}} = \text{mg/kg dose}$$

As this is related to lean body weight, the dose should be reduced by 25% for an obese child. Similarly if the child is oedematous, doses based on the above calculation may also require to be lowered. Phenobarbitone, phenytoin and carbamazepine are enzyme inducers which may increase the metabolism of other lipid soluble drugs and, therefore, their dosage requirement. Penicillins and cephalosporins require high peak levels and as they have short half-lives (about 1 hour), doses at the upper range are recommended. Infants are very sensitive to the pharmacological effects of opiate analgesics and doses at lower range are initially advised. Calculations of dosage for school children are better based on a percentage method assuming an adult of 65 kg body weight with a 1.76 m^2 surface area as follows:

$$\frac{\text{Surface area of child (m}^2)}{1.76 \text{ m}^2} \times 100 = \% \text{ of adult dose}$$

A rough guide is given below:

Approx. age (years)	Weight (kg)	Surface area (m^2)	% of adult dose
5	18	0.74	40
7	23	0.87	50
10	32	1.09	60
12	40	1.27	75
14	45	1.38	80

Both systems for paediatric dosage calculation assume normal renal and hepatic function. Clearly adjustments will be required depending on the clinical pharmacology of the individual drug if the child has documented hepatic cirrhosis or chronic renal failure. Prior to handing over the prescription, it is prudent to compare the calculated daily dose with the normal adult dose to ensure that a decimal point error

7

Cautions

223

has not been made. Liquid preparations are most often used in children as these are absorbed more rapidly than tablets or capsules. Sucrose-based preparations should be avoided wherever possible if chronic therapy is considered. Rectal drug administration is not recommended except for diazepam in epilepsy. If parenteral therapy is indicated the intravenous route should be preferred as it is less painful and more likely to be effective. Drugs are probably best administered at approximately half-life intervals and, as a general rule, the half-life is longer in babies and shorter in pre-adolescent children than in the adult. Adjustment in dosage frequency may also be made according to response, e.g. theophylline in asthma or adverse effects, e.g. sedation with carbamazepine. Therapeutic drug monitoring can be employed in children although the assumption of a similar therapeutic range to the adult may not be justified. Treatment is continued for similar periods in children as adults for most acute conditions and chronic therapy should be contemplated only where essential, e.g. asthma, epilepsy.

7

Cautions

PRESCRIBING IN PREGNANCY

The use of drugs in pregnancy should be confined to those essential to maternal and fetal health and well-being. Although all drugs have the potential for adverse effects, situations in pregnancy do arise where drug therapy is indicated and there are a number of agents which have withstood the test of time and can be regarded as 'safe':

NAUSEA	— small frequent dry meals
	— antihistamine, e.g. promethazine if necessary
HEARTBURN	— advice on posture
	— aluminum hydroxide/magnesium trisilicate mixtures e.g. Maalox, Dijex
CONSTIPATION	— high roughage diet
	— extra bran
	— suppository if essential, e.g. bisacodyl
INFECTION	— penicillin, e.g. ampicillin, amoxycillin
	— cephalosporin, e.g. cephalexin, cephradine
	— erythromycin
VAGINAL DISCHARGE	— miconazole pessaries (monilia)
	— metronidazole (trichomonas)
BACKACHE	— paracetamol (may require to be given 4 hourly)
	— non steroidal anti-inflammatory, e.g. ibuprofen, naproxen, piroxicam only if essential
MIGRAINE	— paracetamol
	— metoclopramide parenterally if necessary
INSOMNIA	— hot milk prior to retiring
	— avoid benzodiazepines
HYPERTENSION	— methyldopa
	— beta blockers, e.g. atenolol
	— hydralazine
TUBERCULOSIS	— rifampicin, isoniazid and ethambutol
MALARIA	— prophylaxis and treatment as appropriate. Risk of malaria greater than fear of teratogenesis
DIABETES MELLITUS	— insulin
THREADWORMS	— piperazine
ANTICOAGULATION	— heparin
	— warfarin in mid-trimester if essential
EPILEPSY	— do not change drugs during pregnancy
	— carbamazepine probably least teratogenic
THYROTOXICOSIS	— carbimazole (smallest controlling dose)
	— propranolol

7

Cautions

TERATOGENESIS

All drugs taken regularly, with the exception of heparin, will cross the placenta and establish equilibrium plasma levels between mother and fetus. Water soluble drugs will do this more slowly than lipid soluble compounds. In the 2nd and 3rd trimesters damage may occur to formed organs, e.g. ototoxicity with streptomycin. In the 1st trimester, particularly in the first 8 weeks of life, damage to developing organs may result in teratogenesis. For a drug to be a proven teratogen, it must cause fetal malformations in a greater proportion of infants than will occur in a similar group of women not taking the drug (1–2% overall) e.g. 6% for phenytoin; or result in a very unusual deformity, e.g. phocomelia with thalidomide.

Teratogens usually produce a consistent pattern of deformity. As it is impossible to prove both scientifically or legally that an individual drug did *not* produce a fetal abnormality in a susceptible patient, e.g. with Debendox, drugs should be prescribed in early pregnancy only when clinically essential. Well-documented examples of teratogenesis are listed below:

Drug	Abnormalities
BARBITURATES	Multiple, especially CNS
CYTOTOXIC AGENTS	Multiple
DIAZEPAM	Orofacial clefts
ETHANOL	Facial abnormalities, mental retardation, multiple organ malformations
LITHIUM	Congenital heart disease
LIVE VACCINES	Multiple
PHENYTOIN	Orofacial clefts, congenital heart disease
SODIUM VALPROATE	Neural tube defects
STILBOESTROL	Genital tract abnormalities
TETRACYCLINES	Multiple, especially bone and teeth
WARFARIN	Nasal hypoplasia, stippled epiphyses, CNS defects

There are a smaller number of drug-related problems with fully-formed organs.

Drug	Abnormalities
AMINOGLYCOSIDE ANTIBIOTICS	Ototoxicity
ANTITHYROID DRUGS	Goitre and hypothyroidism
INDOMETHACIN (AND OTHER NSAIDs)	Premature closure of ductus arteriosus
TETRACYCLINES	Staining of teeth, impaired dentition

DRUGS AND BREAST FEEDING

Most drugs will pass into breast milk to a greater or lesser extent. Lipid soluble drugs pass into milk more quickly than water soluble drugs but if the drug is being taken chronically this differentiation is less relevant. Small water soluble molecules such as ethanol pass very readily into milk. Basic drugs tend to concentrate in milk whereas acidic drugs have a milk/plasma ratio of < 1. Highly protein bound drugs such as warfarin cause fewer problems since only the small proportion of unbound drug is free to cross biological membranes. If the mother is on regular drug therapy, the baby will also receive regular oral doses of drug. Ideally, feeding should take place just before the mother takes her medication.

Possible side-effects can be split into two categories: (1) idiosyncratic reactions such as hepatitis with isoniazid will be very rare occurring in 1/1000–1/10 000 instances but will require only very small amounts of drug; (2) with more substantial amounts, predictable adverse reactions may be seen but the significance of these is often difficult to assess in a new-born infant. Whether beta blockade is harmful to a healthy neonate, for example, is debatable. Well documented adverse effects of drugs in breast-fed infants are not common and are summarised below. Many of these are single case reports and will not occur in the majority of exposed infants.

Mother's drug	Effect on baby
AMANTADINE	Rash, vomiting, urinary retention
AMPICILLIN	Rash, diarrhoea, candidosis
ANTHRAQUINONE LAXATIVES	Diarrhoea
ANTITHYROID DRUGS	Goitre, agranulocytosis
ASPIRIN	Rash, impaired platelet function
ATROPINE	Mydriasis, tachycardia, constipation
BARBITURATES	Drowsiness, blood dyscrasias
BROMIDES	Rash, drowsiness
CAFFEINE	Irritability
CARISOPRODOL	Drowsiness, diarrhoea
CHLORAL HYDRATE	Drowsiness
CHLORAMPHENICOL	Bone marrow depression
CHLORPROMAZINE	Drowsiness
CLONIDINE	Bradycardia
CYCLOPHOSPHAMIDE	Bone marrow depression
DAPSONE	Pigmentation, jaundice, haemolysis
DIAZEPAM	Lethargy, weight loss
DICHLORALPHENAZONE	Drowsiness
EPHEDRINE	Irritability, insomnia
ERGOTAMINE	Ergotism
ETHANOL	Sedation
HEROIN	Addiction
INDOMETHACIN	Seizures

7

Cautions

IODIDES	Goitre
LITHIUM	Hypotonia, hypothermia, cyanosis
MEPROBAMATE	Lethargy
METHADONE	Addiction
METRONIDAZOLE	Unpleasant taste
MORPHINE	Addiction
NALIDIXIC ACID	Haemolytic anaemia
ORAL CONTRACEPTIVES	Gynaecomastia, vaginal epithelial proliferation
PHENINDIONE	Bleeding
PHENOLPHTHALEIN	Rash, diarrhoea
PHENYTOIN	Methaemoglobinaemia, vomiting, tremor
PRIMIDONE	Sedation
RESERPINE	Nasal stuffiness, lethargy, diarrhoea, galactorrhoea
SMOKING (HEAVY)	Restlessness
SULPHONAMIDES	Rash, jaundice, haemolytic anaemia
TETRACYCLINES	Mottling of teeth, impaired dentition
THEOPHYLLINE	Irritability, insomnia
VITAMIN D	Hypercalcaemia

Despite these reports, few drugs are actually contraindicated for the breast-fed infant although some others must be used with caution.

Drugs contraindicated if breast feeding

Amantadine	Gold salts
Androgens	Iodides
Antithyroid drugs	Lithium
Atropine	Oestrogens (high dose)
Bromides	Opiates (addicts)
Bromocriptine	Phenindione
Carisoprodol	Phenylbutazone
Chloramphenicol	Radiopharmaceuticals
Cytotoxic agents	Tetracyclines
Ergotamine	Vitamins A and D (high dose)

Drugs requiring caution if breast feeding

Aminoglycosides	Ethanol
Anthraquinone laxatives	Ethosuximide
Aspirin (high dose)	Meprobamate
Barbiturates	Methyldopa
Carbamazepine	Metronidazole
Chloral hydrate	Nalidixic acid
Cimetidine	Oral contraceptives
Clonidine	Phenytoin
Clorazepate	Primidone
Codeine	Quinidine
Corticosteroids	Reserpine
Dapsone	Sulphasalazine
Dextropropoxyphene	Sulphonamides
Disopyramide	Sulphonylureas
Diuretics	Theophylline

Cautions

Several drugs may affect milk production:

Reduce	Increase
Bromocriptine	Methyldopa
Cyproheptadine	Metoclopramide
Diuretics	Neuroleptics, e.g. chlorpromazine
Ethanol	
Oestrogens	

A common sense approach regarding breast feeding is clearly warranted. Nursing mothers should avoid drugs either self-medicated or prescribed as far as is reasonable. However, the benefits of breast feeding to mother and child should not be needlessly sacrificed. Full discussion with the family and a watching brief by mother and doctor will usually result in a satisfactory outcome.

7

Cautions

DRUGS IN HEPATIC DISEASE

Most drugs are lipid-soluble and must be metabolised to more water soluble molecules prior to excretion in the bile and/or urine. Drug metabolism is only impaired to a clinically significant extent where there is severe liver disease, e.g. acute viral hepatitis, active chronic hepatitis, cirrhosis and some patients with severe congestive cardiac failure. As a general rule oxidation reactions are much more affected than conjugating mechanisms and standard doses of oxidised drugs with a narrow therapeutic ratio should be reduced by 50% in patients with histologically-proven hepatic cirrhosis. A lower dose may be required if there are signs of jaundice, hypoalbuminaemia, clotting disturbance and ascites. Drugs metabolised largely by conjugation can be given in the usual dose unless clinical signs of hepatic decompensation supervene. The oral bioavailability of drugs with a substantial, i.e. greater than 50%, first pass metabolism may be increased several fold in cirrhotic patients and these drugs should be used with extreme caution in patients with severe liver disease. Decompensated cirrhotics may be precipitated into pre-coma by sedative drugs e.g. opioid analgesics, benzodiazepines, neuroleptics, antidepressants.

Partial list of groups of drugs inactivated in the liver

Drug group	Examples
ANAESTHETICS	Halothane
ANTIARRHYTHMICS	Lignocaine
	Quinidine
	Verapamil
ANTIBIOTICS	Chloramphenicol
	Doxycycline
	Rifampicin
ANTICOAGULANTS	Warfarin
ANTICONVULSANTS	Carbamazepine
	Phenobarbitone
	Phenytoin
	Primidone
	Sodium valproate
ANTIHYPERTENSIVES	Hydralazine
	Labetalol
	Methyldopa
	Metoprolol
	Oxprenolol
	Prazosin
	Propranolol
ANTIHISTAMINES	Diphenhydramine
BRONCHODILATORS	Theophylline
HYPOGLYCAEMICS	Glibenclamide
	Tolbutamide
NARCOTIC ANALGESICS	Morphine
	Pethidine

NEUROLEPTICS	Chlorpromazine
	Haloperidol
SEDATIVES	Chlordiazepoxide
	Diazepam
	Glutethimide
	Meprobamate
STEROIDS	Dexamethasone
	Hydrocortisone
	Oral contraceptives
	Prednisolone
THYROID HORMONES	Thyroxine

Drugs undergoing substantial first pass metabolism

Cardiac
Glyceryl trinitrate
Hydralazine
Indoramin
Isoprenaline
Isosorbide dinitrate
Labatolol
Lignocaine
Metoprolol
Prazosin
Propranolol
Verapamil

Respiratory
Salbutamol
Terbutaline

Neurological
Dihydroergotamine
Levodopa
Neostigmine

Analgesic
Aspirin
Codeine
Dextropropoxyphene
Meptazinol
Morphine
Pentazocine
Pethidine

Psychiatric
Amitriptyline
Chlormethiazole
Chlorpromazine
Doxepin
Imipramine
Methylphenidate
Nortriptyline

Cytotoxic
Fluorouracil
Mercaptopurine

Others
Domperidone
Oral contraceptives
Praziquantel

7

Cautions

DRUGS IN RENAL FAILURE

A small number of water-soluble drugs are excreted largely unchanged by the kidney. Dosages of these drugs may require to be reduced in patients with renal disease, most often according to the reduction in creatinine clearance. An alternative option is to increase the dosage interval if a high trough concentration is to be avoided, e.g. with aminoglycoside antibiotics. Drugs with a high therapeutic index such as penicillin will not require much change in dosage while with more toxic drugs such as gentamicin, digoxin and lithium close regulation of dose is essential with therapeutic monitoring of circulating drug levels. Drugs which are primarily metabolised in the liver rarely require dosage reduction in renal failure. A problem may arise when a drug is partly metabolised and partly excreted unchanged such as chlorpropamide and procainamide. In such situations careful supervision of the effect of the drug is required and often dosage reduction is necessary if either renal or hepatic function is impaired. A partial list of drugs excreted largely unchanged by the kidney is given below. When starting therapy, the loading dose need not be adjusted.

Drugs excreted largely unchanged by the kidney

Acetohexamide
Acyclovir
Amantadine
Aminoglycosides
Atenolol
Baclofen
Bethanidine
Bleomycin
Bretylium
Bumetanide
Cephalosporins
Chloroquine
Chlorothiazide
Chlorpropamide
Cimetidine
Cisplatin

Digoxin
Ethambutol
Flucytosine
Frusemide
Guanethidine
Hyoscine
Lithium
Metformin
Methotrexate
Nadolol
Penicillins
Pirenzepine
Procainamide
Ranitidine
Sotalol
Tetracycline

7

Cautions

PRESCRIBING FOR THE ELDERLY

The major constraint in prescribing for the elderly is the risk of
adverse reactions. As the elderly are more likely to receive multiple
drugs, interactions are also more frequent. Knowledge of the
pharmacology of the individual drugs prescribed is helpful in view of
the multiple alterations in drug handling and response occurring as a
consequence of ageing.

Alterations in drug handling and response in the elderly

ABSORPTION	Unaltered
DISTRIBUTION	Lipid soluble drugs
	— lower circulating levels
	— higher volume of distribution
	Water soluble drugs
	— higher circulating levels
	— lower volume of distribution
	Reduced protein binding
METABOLISM	Reduced oxidative capacity
	Reduced first pass metabolism
	Normal conjugating processes
	Decreased inducibility
RENAL EXCRETION	Lipid soluble drugs — largely unaffected
	Water soluble drugs — reduced elimination
RECEPTORS	Increased sensitivity — warfarin, benzodiazepines
	Reduced numbers — beta blockers
HOMOEOSTASIS	Impaired
	— postural hypotension (diuretics)
	— confusion (sedatives)
	— hypothermia (neuroleptics)
MULTIPLE DISEASE STATES	Common
DRUG INTERACTIONS	More likely
COMPLIANCE	Poor

As body water is decreased and body fat increased, changes in
distribution are responsible for lower circulating levels of lipid soluble
drugs and relatively higher concentrations of water soluble drugs
than in younger patients. Although reduced compared to younger
people, impaired hepatic oxidative metabolism is not a common
cause of major problems in the elderly. The exception may be with
those drugs with a high first pass metabolism as increased
bioavailability may produce a substantially higher peak and steady-
state concentration than expected. Reduced renal excretion of water
soluble drugs is most important if the drug has a narrow therapeutic
ratio, e.g. digoxin, lithium. Serum creatinine in the elderly always

7

Cautions

overestimates creatinine clearance as creatinine production falls with age. Receptor sensitivity may be increased but receptor numbers may be reduced and so drug response in the elderly is often unpredictable. Impairment of homeostasis may be responsible for postural hypotensive effects with a variety of drugs, e.g. diuretics, nitrates, tricyclic antidepressants. In addition, multiple disease states are common and compliance is often poor. Some common problems with individual drug groups are listed below.

Common adverse drug effects in the elderly

Drug	Problems
ANTICHOLINERGICS	Dry mouth, glaucoma, constipation, hallucinations
ANTIHYPERTENSIVES	Postural hypotension
BENZODIAZEPINES	Daytime drowsiness, confusion, falls, dependence
BETA BLOCKERS	Fatigue, cold extremities, bronchospasm, bradycardia, cardiac failure
CIMETIDINE	Confusion
CORTICOSTEROIDS	Cataracts, osteoporotic fractures
DIGOXIN	Confusion, nausea, arrhythmias
DIURETICS	Postural hypotension, hypokalaemia, gout, glucose intolerance
LEVODOPA	Confusion, hypotension, nausea
LITHIUM	Toxicity
NEUROLEPTICS	Sedation, postural hypotension, hypothermia, extrapyramidal reactions, tardive dyskinesia
NON-STEROIDAL ANTIINFLAMMATORIES	Dyspepsia, gastrointestinal bleeding, confusion, fluid retention, hypertension
OPIATES	Increased sensitivity
ORAL HYPOGLYCAEMICS	Nocturnal hypoglycaemia
TETRACYCLINES	Renal failure
TRICYCLIC ANTIDEPRESSANTS	Sedation, postural hypotension, anticholinergic effects
WARFARIN	Increased sensitivity

Probably the biggest problem in rationalising prescribing for the elderly is the inconsistency of the alterations in drug handling or response between individual patients. The elderly are not an homogeneous population and chronological age may not be a true reflection of biological age. The presence of disease states affecting particularly the organs of drug elimination, namely the liver and kidney, may be a further confounding factor. A number of simple rules of prescribing for the elderly should be followed.

1. Only prescribe when essential.
2. Choose a drug with the widest therapeutic ratio.
3. Know its pharmacology.
4. Start at a low dosage.
5. Give as few daily doses as possible.
6. Consider possible interactions before introducing new drug.
7. Monitor response and possible toxicity soon after introduction.
8. Avoid combination preparations.
9. Resist new drugs.
10. Review treatment schedule regularly.
11. Beware repeat prescribing.

NEW DRUGS

When the regulatory drug authority releases a new drug for clinical use, it has concerned itself with a number of important aspects. Firstly the drug must be pharmacologically effective. It must fulfil certain criteria of safety in animal testing and in early pre-marketing trials in man — usually in around 1000 patients. Care is taken to ensure that the dosage regimen suggested reflects its pharmacokinetics — usually in young healthy volunteers. Finally the quality of the formulation is guaranteed. What is not considered is comparison with existing similar agents both regarding efficacy and safety, i.e. there is no assessment of the overall need for the drug. Thus new beta blockers, benzodiazepine hypnotics, non-steroidal anti-inflammatory agents and oral hypoglycaemics are released every year.

Clearly it is the role of the pharmaceutical industry which is now almost wholly responsible for the development of new chemical entities to promote these to the prescriber. As each successful new product is estimated to cost around £90 million from synthesis to licensing and this process takes more than 10 years to complete, it is not surprising that the company is anxious to recoup financially for this and other less successful compounds. The situation is compounded by the relatively short period for which the patent for a new drug is guaranteed, namely 16 years. As a result marketing is often aggressive.

For a new drug to find its place in the therapeutic armamentarium, the results of a number of controlled clinical trials are required. Ideally the drug should be compared to a placebo and then to its major competitors. For ethical reasons, the former studies are rarely now carried out. Trials should be double-blind and randomised to avoid bias. The entry criteria must be clearly defined and enough patients included to detect a difference. This is where placebo trials are particularly valuable. If too few patients are included, the drug may be shown to be no more effective than a placebo. If too few patients are enrolled in a comparative trial with a competitor, the study may conclude that it is as effective as the standard available drug. Comparisons should be made between comparable doses as this also can lead to false enthusiasm for the new agent. Care should also be taken to scrutinise the results of a study to ensure that the advantages shown are of biological as well as statistical significance. A small consistent fall in blood pressure may produce very impressive statistics but be clinically irrelevant.

Similarly, clinical trials should be as rigorous in assessing adverse reactions as pharmacological effects. Close scrutiny of large scale studies should provide information on patient withdrawals as well as the incidence of subjective side-effects. The production of severe idiosyncratic drug reactions such as aplastic anaemia and hepatotoxicity can only be identified when substantial numbers of patients have received the drug chronically. This may be accomplished by large post-marketing surveillance studies. The incidence of hepatotoxicity with benoxaprofen was around 1:5000 patients and was only detected after a substantial number of fatalities.

There seems little need to prescribe a new drug if a number of well-proven alternatives are available. Theoretical marketing claims must be compared to established advantages following controlled trials and extensive post-marketing surveillance. If a major advantage is claimed and there seems to be evidence to support it then the drug may be prescribed but close follow-up must be undertaken both for therapeutic efficacy and toxic effects. Some examples of such claims are shown below. Wherever possible, objective evidence of benefit should be sought. All side-effects, however minor, should be reported to the appropriate regulatory authority. Patients receiving new drugs should be followed up for some years as long-term toxicity, e.g. mucocutaneous syndrome with practolol may not be apparent for some substantial time. As a general rule, only specialists should prescribe new drugs until proper clinical assessment has taken place.

Reasons for prescribing a new drug

1. No existing drug for the disease, e.g. acyclovir.
2. More effective than alternatives, e.g. H_2 antagonists.
3. Advantageous side effect profile, e.g. terfenadine.
4. Fewer adverse drug reactions and interactions, e.g. ranitidine.
5. Better pharmacokinetic profile, e.g. isosorbide mononitrate.
6. Equivalent but cheaper, e.g. ?

7

Cautions

COMBINATION PREPARATIONS

It is tempting to endeavour to improve compliance by prescribing a preparation containing two or more drugs. This can be particularly successful when the components have synergistic properties, e.g. co-trimoxazole, oral contraceptive pill. The major disadvantage to this approach is that the amounts of both drugs are fixed and, therefore, inflexible. It is important to ensure that the bioavailability of both components has been shown to be equivalent when given alone and in the combined form, that the doses of both are appropriate and that the duration of effect of each is similar. The patient must clearly benefit from both components in the formulation and consideration of the likely adverse effects must be taken into account. The effect of disease or old age on the pharmacokinetics and pharmacodynamics of each drug may differ and this will increase the possibility of toxicity. Cost may also be a factor. It is surprisingly easy to forget that a new product contains two pharmacological ingredients and prescribe a second drug with similar properties to one of the components of the combination, e.g. diuretic/beta blocker combination and another diuretic. Certainly if a single combination tablet does not produce a satisfactory response without unacceptable side-effects, the combination might best be discarded. There is no advantage in compliance in taking a combined preparation once a day rather than its individual components also only once daily. Combination preparations are clearly here to stay and require close and careful monitoring of efficacy and toxicity.

7

Cautions

THERAPEUTIC DRUG MONITORING

For a few drugs, plasma levels are helpful in predicting clinical response and potential toxicity. These are drugs with a narrow therapeutic ratio which are often implicated in the production of adverse effects and interactions. Peak concentrations can be obtained around 1-2 hours after the dose and trough levels occur shortly after a dose during the lag time before absorption begins. When prescribing for an individual patient, the therapeutic range can never be more than a guide as there are patients who respond satisfactorily to low drug concentrations whereas others require concentrations well above it. Similarly some patients exhibit toxicity within the range whereas others tolerate very high concentrations. A knowledge of the level, however, does allow the prescriber to appreciate whether the patient is compliant, whether suspected toxicity is confirmed or whether there is substantial leeway for increasing the dose. Most biochemistry departments now provide a drug assay service although the clinical value to the prescriber varies for individual drugs. A common selection of available assays with the appropriate 'therapeutic ranges' is shown below. Monitoring is essential for phenytoin, lithium, gentamicin and tobramycin; useful for carbamazepine, phenobarbitone, procainamide, lignocaine, digoxin, mexilitene and theophylline; and of limited value for the rest.

Target ranges

	Drug	Metric	Molar
†	Carbamazepine	4–10 mg/l	17–42 µmol/l
†	Digoxin	0.8–2 ng/ml	1–2.6 nmol/l
	Disopyramide	2.4–7 mg/l	7.1–20.6 µmol/l
	Ethosuximide	40–100 mg/l	283–708 µmol/l
*	Gentamicin — peak	5–10 mg/l	10.8–21.6 µmol/l
	— trough	< 2 mg/l	< 4.3 µmol/l
†	Lignocaine	1.5–5 mg/l	6.4–21.3 µmol/l
*	Lithium	4–11 mg/l	0.6–1.6 mmol/l
†	Mexiletine	0.75–2 mg/l	4.2–11.1 mmol/l
†	Phenobarbitone	10–40 mg/l	43–172 µmol/l
	(febrile convulsions)	(15–20 mg/l)	(65–86 µmol/l)
*	Phenytoin	10–20 mg/l	40–80 µmol/l
	Primidone	5–12 mg/l	23–55 µmol/l
†	Procainamide	4–10 mg/l	17–42.5 µmol/l
	Quinidine	2–5.5 mg/l	6.2–16.9 µmol/l
	Sodium valproate	50–100 mg/l	347–693 µmol/l
†	Theophylline	10–20 mg/l	55.5–111 µmol/l
*	Tobramycin — peak	5–10 mg/l	11–21 µmol/l
	— trough	< 2 mg/l	< 4.3 µmol/l

* Essential;   † Useful.

7

Cautions

COMPLIANCE

Thirty per cent of patients fail to take the prescribed doses of their drugs at the correct time. Good compliance cannot be assumed and poor compliers when identified require careful and skillful handling. A four stage plan for such patients is often helpful.

1. Identify the reasons for defaulting therapy;
   such as — fear of becoming drug dependent,
       e.g. anticonvulsants
   — delayed onset of drug action, e.g. tricyclic antidepressants
   — patient becoming asymptomatic, e.g. antibiotic
   — development of adverse effect, e.g. sexual problem

2. Educate the patient at his own socio-economic level;
   discuss — purpose of treatment, e.g. epilepsy, diabetes, asthma
   — the role of each drug, e.g. symptomatic or prophylactic
   — expected side-effects, e.g. headache with a nitrate, fatigue with a beta blocker, sedation with an antidepressant
   — probable duration of therapy, e.g. acute, chronic, life-long
   — supplementary leaflets as available

3. Devise a treatment plan to fit with the patient's life style;
   take into consideration — unsocial working hours
   — minimal number of drugs required
   — frequency of administration, e.g. twice rather than three times daily
   — provision of a drug card
   — supervision of tablet taking by relative or friend

4. Monitor compliance and response to treatment;
   see the patient regularly and — take measurements when possible,
   e.g. BP, peak flow, pulse, angina diary, seizure frequency chart
   — ask about specific side-effects, e.g. fatigue with beta blockers, sedation with antidepressants, sexual difficulties with an antihypertensive
   — arrange to see the medicine bottles at each visit
   — organise a relative to check adherence to treatment schedule

EFFECT OF DRUGS ON LABORATORY VALUES

Laboratory testing plays an important role in clinical practice. Drug treatment can, not surprisingly, affect the results of a number of common biochemical and haematological investigations. This may be due to a pharmacological effect of the drug, e.g. hyperuricaemia with thiazide diuretics or drug-induced disease, e.g. cholestatic jaundice with chlorpromazine. The difference between these effects may be purely quantitative. Thus, although most patients receiving thiazide diuretics have asymptomatic hyperuricaemia, a few do develop acute gout. On other occasions, the drug or metabolite may interfere with the measurement requested. Thus, methyldopa, itself a catecholamine precursor, may produce a false positive test for urinary catecholamine metabolites in a patient suspected of having a phaeochromocytoma. Unfortunately drugs may affect one method of performing a given laboratory test and have no effect on another. The following is a short list of drug-related effects on laboratory values. In a patient such changes should not be assumed to be a laboratory artefact and drug-induced disease must be excluded.

A. Blood tests

Raised serum amylase

Asparaginase
Azathioprine
Corticosteroids
Cyproheptadine
Frusemide
Methyldopa
Opiate analgesics
Oral contraceptives
Procainamide
Rifampicin
Sodium valproate
Sulphasalazine
Tetracycline
Thiazide diuretics

Raised serum alanine aminotransferase (ALT)

Allopurinol
Anabolic steroids
Azathioprine
Erythromycin
Ethanol
Halothane
Isoniazid
Levodopa
Methyldopa
Nitrofurantoin
Oral contraceptives
Phenothiazines
Sodium valproate

Raised serum alkaline phosphatase

Anabolic steroids
Benzodiazepines
Disulfiram
Erythromycin
Ethanol
Methyldopa
Nitrofurantoin
Oral contraceptives
Phenothiazines
Phenytoin

7

Cautions

Raised serum bilirubin

Allopurinol
Anabolic steroids
Azathioprine
Beta blockers
Disulfiram
Erythromycin

Ethanol
Levodopa
Methyldopa
Phenothiazines
Rifampicin

Serum calcium

Rise
Anabolic steroids
Lithium
Oral contraceptives

Fall
Carbamazepine
Cimetidine
Phenobarbitone
Phenytoin

Blood glucose

Rise
Acetazolamide
Beta agonists
Corticosteroids
Diazoxide
Ethacrynic acid
Frusemide
Isoniazid
Levodopa
Metronidazole
Nalidixic acid
Oral contraceptives
Phenothiazines
Phenytoin
Prazosin
Thiazide diuretics

Fall
Anabolic steroids
Aspirin
Beta blockers
Clofibrate
Dextropropoxyphene
Ethanol
Guanethidine
Monoamine oxidase inhibitors

Serum potassium

Rise
Amiloride
Captopril
Cytotoxic agents
Isoniazid
Potassium supplements
Spironolactone
Triamterene

Fall
Amphotericin
Bumetanide
Carbenicillin
Carbenoxolone
Corticosteroids
Frusemide
Insulin
Laxative abuse
Levodopa
Salicylate overdose
Thiazide diuretics

Cautions

7

Raised serum prolactin

Cimetidine
Haloperidol
Methyldopa
Metoclopramide

Monoamine oxidase inhibitors
Phenothiazines
Reserpine

Circulating thyroid hormones

Rise
Amiodarone
Oestrogens
Oral contraceptives

Fall
Amiodarone
Anabolic steroids
Beta blockers
Lithium
Non-steroidal antiinflammatories

Raised serum triglycerides

Corticosteroids
Ethanol

Oestrogens
Oral contraceptives

Raised serum uric acid

Anabolic steroids
Bumetanide
Cytotoxic agents
Diazoxide
Ethacrynic acid
Ethambutol

Ethanol
Frusemide
Levodopa
Pyrazinamide
Thiazide diuretics
Triamterene

Raised serum urea

Aminoglycosides
Corticosteroids
Diuretics

Salicylates
Tetracyclines

B. Urine tests

Raised urinary catecholamines and metabolites
(Diagnosis of phaeochromocytoma)

Levodopa
Methyldopa
Paracetamol
Phenothiazines

Quinidine
Reserpine
Tetracycline
Theophylline

Increased urinary glucose

as for blood glucose and
Aminoglycosides
Cephalosporins

Chloramphenicol
Probenecid

Cautions

7

FORMULATION, FOOD AND DRUG ABSORPTION

A tablet formulation of a drug will depend on many variables including the diluent, disintegrant and lubricant as well as the size of the granules from which the tablet is compressed, pressure and speed of compression and subsequent storage conditions. Variation in drug response both in terms of therapeutic efficacy and adverse effects may occur with different formulations of the same chemotherapeutic agent. This is one argument for not using generic equivalents. As bioavailability data is now required from manufacturers prior to general release, this problem should not arise with drugs originating in the United Kingdom but may still do with imported 'replicas'. A liquid preparation is often quicker (and more completely) absorbed than an equivalent tablet or capsule. Dissolution of a capsule formulation may be erratic. On occasions substitution of one formulation for another may improve patient acceptability.

As a general rule, absorption of lipid soluble drugs is enhanced in the presence of fatty foods although as these drugs are well absorbed anyway this is unlikely to make much of a difference. Water soluble drugs, whose absorption may be incomplete at best, should be taken on an empty stomach at least 1 hour prior to a meal. A full glass of water taken with a tablet or capsule formulation will enhance dissolution. Drugs for whom better absorption has been demonstrated on an empty stomach are listed below.

Drugs better taken on an empty stomach

Captopril	Methotrexate
Cephalosporins	Penicillins
Digoxin	Propantheline
Dipyridamole	Rifampicin
Erythromycin	Tetracyclines
Isoniazid	

A further factor to be considered is the likelihood of the drug to produce local gastrointestinal irritation. These preparations should be taken with food to prevent or reduce adverse local effects. Pro-drugs can also be used to overcome such a problem. Thus ampicillin esters (talampicillin, bacampicillin and pivampicillin), which are hydrolysed to the parent drug in the gut wall, are said to produce a lower incidence of diarrhoea and may have improved ampicillin bioavailability. However, they are also substantially more expensive. The non-steroidal anti-inflammatory agent, fenbufen is metabolised to its active form in the liver and may, therefore, exhibit a lower incidence of local gastrointestinal effects than its competitors. The drugs listed below are better taken with food.

Drugs producing local gastrointestinal irritation

Allopurinol
Amiodarone
Baclofen
Bromocriptine
Carbamazepine
Chlorpropamide
Cinnarizine
Clofibrate
Co-trimoxazole
Disopyramide
Emepromium bromide
Flavoxate
Levodopa
Lidoflazine
Lithium
Metformin
Methysergide
Metronidazole
Nalidixic acid
Nitrofurantoin
Non-steroidal anti-inflammatory agents
Potassium salts
Procyclidine
Quinine
Reserpine
Sodium fusidate
Sodium valproate
Sulphasalazine
Sulphinpyrazone
Sulphonamides
Theophylline
Tolbutamide
Triamterene
Viloxazine
Zinc sulphate

The effect of food on drug absorption is a complex issue. Most drugs are absorbed perfectly adequately when given with food with less chance of producing gastrointestinal intolerance. A few water soluble drugs and lipid soluble antibiotics represent exceptions. However, clearly if a drug is not adequately absorbed it is unlikely to produce a therapeutic effect.

SHELF LIFE

Decomposition reactions of formulated products may vary substantially. Prediction of the extent is, therefore, impractical and a set of arbitrary rules must be adhered to. 'Normal storage conditions' depends on the country of origin of the drug product and the climate in the country of use. Unless the storage conditions are defined precisely on the container, allowances must be made for environmental variation. The following list is a guide to typical shelf lives. Although some deterioration may take place, the product may retain acceptable pharmacological activity for much longer.

Product	Duration	Comments
TABLETS AND CAPSULES	3–5 years	If stored in a cool dry place
except antibiotics	2–3 years	Potency loss is a function of time
glyceryl trinitrate	1–2 months	May lose effect in patient's pocket
MIXTURES	3–12 months	Unopened
	1–3 months	Once opened
except diamorphine	2–4 weeks	Converts to morphine
antibiotics	7–14 days	After reconstitution
SYRUPS	1–3 years	High osmolarity inhibits bacterial but not fungal growth
EYE DROPS	1–2 years	Unopened
	2–4 weeks	Once opened
EMULSIONS	Variable	May cream, crack or coagulate
CREAMS	1–3 years	Unopened tubes
	2 weeks	Once opened
OINTMENTS	1–3 years	Unopened tubes
	4–8 weeks	Once opened
SUPPOSITORIES	1–3 months	If not hermetically sealed, glycerin bases can absorb water
INJECTION ADDITIVES	24–72 hours	If added aseptically and stored in refrigerator
except ampicillin	6 hours	Breaks down in dextrose solutions
MULTIDOSE VIALS	1–3 years	If a preservative is included
LIVE VACCINES	1–12 months	Avoid freezing

Proprietary– Generic Drugs

Abicol*
RESERPINE/BENDROFLUAZIDE

ACEBUTOLOL
Sectral

Acepril
CAPTOPRIL

Achromycin
TETRACYCLINE OINTMENT

ACETOHEXAMIDE
Diamox

ACETYL SALICYLIC ACID
see ASPIRIN

Actidil
TRIPROLIDINE

ACTINOMYCIN D
Cosmegen

Acupan
NEFOPAM

ACYCLOVIR
Zovirax

Adalat
NIFEDIPINE

Adcortyl
TRIAMCINOLONE

Adriamycin
DOXORUBICIN

Aerosporin
POLYMIXIN

Agarol*
LIQUID PARAFFIN/PHENOLPHTHALEIN

Alcobon
FLUCYTOSINE

Aldactone
SPIRONOLACTONE

Aldomet
METHYLDOPA

Alexan
CYTARABINE

Alkeran
MELPHALAN

Allegron
NORTRIPTYLINE

ALLOPURINOL
Aluline, Caplenal, Zyloric

Alophen*
BELLADONNA/PHENOLPHTHALEIN/ ALOIN/IPECACUANHA

ALPRAZOLAM
Xanax

Alrheumat
KETOPROFEN

Aludrox*
ALUMINIUM/MAGNESIUM

Aluline
ALLOPURINOL

Alunex
CHLORPHENIRAMINE

ALUMINIUM/MAGNESIUM
Aludrox*, Dijex*, Gelusil*, Polycrol*, Polycrol Forte*, Prodexin*, Siloxyl*, Topal*

Footnote: The generic names for drugs are given in capitals. * Denotes items that are combination products.

Alupent	ORCIPRENALINE
Alupram	DIAZEPAM
Aluzine	FRUSEMIDE
AMANTADINE	Symmetrel
Amfipen	AMPICILLIN
AMIKACIN	Amikin
Amikin	AMIKACIN
AMILORIDE	Midamor, Frumil*
AMINOGLUTETHIMIDE	Orimeten
AMINOPHYLLINE	Phyllocontin
AMIODARONE	Cordarone X
AMITRIPTYLINE	Domical, Lentizol, Tryptizol
AMOXYCILLIN	Amoxyl
Amoxyl	AMOXYCILLIN
AMPHOTERICIN	Fungizone (oral), Fungilin (topical)
AMPICILLIN	Amfipen, Penbritin, Vidopen
Anafranil	CLOMIPRAMINE
Antabuse	DISULFIRAM
ANTAZOLINE	Otrivine-Antistin (with Xylometazoline)
Antepsin	SUCRALFATE
Anthisan	MEPYRAMINE
Anturan	SULPHINPYRAZONE
Anxon	KETAZOLAM
Apresoline	HYDRALAZINE
Aprinox	BENDROFLUAZIDE
Apsifen	IBUPROFEN
Apsin VK	PENICILLIN V
Apsolol	PROPRANOLOL
Apsolox	OXPRENOLOL
Artane	BENZHEXOL
ASCORBIC ACID	Redoxon, Roscorbic
Asmaven	SALBUTAMOL
ASPIRIN	Breoprin, Claridin, Levius, Nu-Seal Aspirin (enteric coated), Solprin
ASTEMIZOLE	Hismanal
ATENOLOL	Tenormin
Atensine	DIAZEPAM
Ativan	LORAZEPAM
Atromid-S	CLOFIBRATE
Atrovent	IPRATROPIUM
Aureomycin	CHLORTETRACYCLINE

Aventyl	NORTRIPTYLINE
Avloclor	CHLOROQUINE
Avomine	PROMETHAZINE
AZAPROPAZONE	Rheumox
AZATHIOPRINE	Imuran
AZATIDINE	Optimine
AZLOCILLIN	Securopen
BACLOFEN	Lioresal
Bactrim	CO-TRIMOXAZOLE
Baratol	INDORAMIN
Baxan	CEFADROXYL
Baycaron	Mefrusemide
Baypen	MEZLOCILLIN
Becloforte	BECLOMETHASONE
BECLOMETHASONE	Becotide, Becloforte
BECLOMETHASONE NASAL SPRAY	Beconase
Beconase	BECLOMETHASONE NASAL SPRAY
Becotide	BECLOMETHASONE
BELLADONNA	Alophen*, Neutradonna*, Carbellon*
Benadryl	DIPHENHYDRAMINE
Bendogen	BETHANIDINE
BENDROFLUAZIDE	Aprinox, Berkozide, Centyl, Neo-NaClex
Benemid	PROBENECID
Benoryl	BENORYLATE
BENORYLATE	Benoryl
Benoxyl	BENZOYL PEROXIDE
BENSERAZIDE/LEVODOPA	Madopar*
BENZHEXOL	Artane
BENZOYL PEROXIDE	Benoxyl
BENZYDAMINE	Difflam
BENZYLPENICILLIN	Crystapen
Berkatens	VERAPAMIL
Berkfurin	NITROFURANTOIN
Berkmycen	OXYTETRACYCLINE
Berkolol	PROPRANOLOL
Berkozide	BENDROFLUAZIDE
Berotec	FENOTEROL
Beta-Cardone	SOTALOL
BETAHISTINE	Serc
Betaloc	METOPROLOL

Proprietary | Generic Drugs

BETAMETHASONE	Bextasol
BETAMETHASONE CREAM/OINTMENT	Betnovate, Diprosone
BETHANIDINE	Bendogen, Esbatal
Betim	TIMOLOL
Betnovate	BETAMETHASONE (topical)
Bextasol	BETAMETHASONE
Bi CNU	CARMUSTINE
Biogastrone	CARBENOXOLONE
BISACODYL	Dulcolax
BISMUTH CHELATE	De-Nol, De-Noltab
Blocadren	TIMOLOL
Bolvidon	MIANSERIN
Bonjela	CHOLINE SALICYLATE
BRAN	Fybranta
Breoprin	ASPIRIN
Bretylate	BRETYLIUM
BRETYLIUM	Bretylate
Bricanyl	TERBUTALINE
Brocadopa	LEVODOPA
BROMAZEPAM	Lexotan
BROMOCRIPTINE	Parlodel
BROMPHENIRAMINE	Dimotane
Bronchodil	REPROTEROL
Brufen	IBUPROFEN
BUDESONIDE	Pulmicort, Rhinocort
BUMETANIDE	Burinex
BUPRENORPHINE	Temgesic
Burinex	BUMETANIDE
Buscopan	HYOSCINE HYDROBROMIDE
BUSULPHAN	Myleran
Butazone	PHENYLBUTAZONE
BUTORPHANOL	Stadol
Calpol	PARACETAMOL (paediatric syrup)
Camcolit	LITHIUM
Canesten	CLOTRIMAZOLE
Caplenal	ALLOPURINOL
Capoten	CAPTOPRIL
CAPTOPRIL	Acepril, Capoten
CARBAMAZEPINE	Tegretol
Carbellon*	BELLADONNA

CARBENICILLIN	Pyopen
CARBENOXOLONE	Biogastrone, Duogastrone
CARBIDOPA/LEVODOPA	Sinemet*, Sinemet Plus*
CARBIMAZOLE	Neo-Mercazole
CARBOXYMETHYL CELLULOSE GEL	Orabase
Cardiacap	PENTAERYTHRITOL TETRANITRATE
Carisoma	CARISOPRODOL
CARISOPRODOL	Carisoma
CARMUSTINE	Bi CNU
Catapres	CLONIDINE (hypertension dose)
Cedocard	ISOSORBIDE DINITRATE
CEFACLOR	Distaclor
CEFADROXYL	Baxan
CEFOTAXIME	Claforan
CEFOXITIN	Mefoxin
CEFSULODIN	Monaspor
CEFUROXIME	Zinacef
Centrax	PRAZEPAM
Centyl	BENDROFLUAZIDE
CEPHALEXIN	Ceporex, Keflex
CEPHALORIDINE	Ceporin
CEPHALOTHIN	Keflin
CEPHAMANDOLE	Kefadol
CEPHAZOLIN	Kefzol
CEPHRADINE	Velosef
Ceporex	CEPHALEXIN
Ceporin	CEPHALORIDINE
Cesamet	NABILONE
Cetiprin	EMEPRONIUM
Chendol	CHENODEOXYCHOLIC ACID
Chenocedon	CHENODEOXYCHOLIC ACID
CHENODEOXYCHOLIC ACID	Chendol, Chenocedon
CHLORAL HYDRATE	Noctec
CHLORAMBUCIL	Leukeran
CHLORAMPHENICOL	Chloromycetin, Kemicetine
CHLORAMPHENICOL EYE PREPARATIONS	Chloromycetin, Sno Phenicol
CHLORDIAZEPOXIDE	Librium
CHLORMETHIAZOLE	Heminevrin
Chloromycetin	CHLORAMPHENICOL
CHLOROQUINE	Avloclor, Nivaquine

CHLOROTHIAZIDE	Saluric
CHLORPHENIRAMINE	Alunex, Piriton
CHLORPROMAZINE	Largactil
CHLORPROPAMIDE	Diabinese, Melitase
CHLORTETRACYCLINE	Aureomycin
CHOLESTYRAMINE	Questran
CHOLINE SALICYLATE	Bonjela
Cidomycin	GENTAMICIN
CIMETIDINE	Tagamet
CINNARIZINE	Stugeron
CISPLATIN	Neoplatin, Platinex
Claforan	CEFOTAXIME
Claridin	ASPIRIN
CLINDAMYCIN	Dalacin C
Clinium	LIDOFLAZINE
Clinoril	SULINDAC
CLOBAZAM	Frisium
CLOBETASOL CREAM/OINTMENT	Dermovate
CLOBETASONE CREAM/OINTMENT	Eumovate
CLOFIBRATE	Atromid-S
Clomid	CLOMIPHENE
CLOMIPHENE	Clomid, Serophene
CLOMIPRAMINE	Anafranil
CLONAZEPAM	Rivotril
CLONIDINE	
hypertension dose	Catapres
migraine dose	Dixarit
CLOPAMIDE	Brinaldix K*, Viskaldix
CLOPENTHIXOL	Clopixol
Clopixol	CLOPENTHIXOL
CLORAZEPATE	Tranxene
CLOTRIMAZOLE	Canesten
CLOXACILLIN	Orbenin
Cobalin	CYNACOBALAMIN
Codelsol	PREDNISOLONE
Colestid	COLESTIPOL
COLESTIPOL	Colestid
Colifoam	HYDROCORTISONE
Colofac	MEBEVERINE
Concordin	PROTRIPTYLINE
Cordarone X	AMIODARONE

Cordilox	VERAPAMIL
Corgard	NADOLOL
Corlan	HYDROCORTISONE
Coro-Nitro Spray	GLYCERYL TRINITRATE
Cortelan	CORTISONE
Cortenema	HYROCORTISONE
CORTISONE	Cortelan, Cortistab
Cortistab	CORTISONE
Cosalgesic*	DEXTROPROPOXYPHENE/ PARACETAMOL
Cosmegen	ACTINOMYCIN D
CO-TRIMOXAZOLE	Bactrim, Laratrim, Septrin
CYANOCOBALAMIN	Cobalin, Cytamen
Crystapen	BENZYLPENICILLIN
Crystapen V	PENICILLIN V
CYCLIZINE	Valoid
CYCLOPHOSPHAMIDE	Endoxana
Cyclo-progynova*	OESTRADIOL/LEVONORGESTREL
CYCLOSPORIN	Sandimmun
CYPROHEPTADINE	Periactin
Cytamen	CYANOCOBALAMIN
CYTARABINE	Alexan, Cytosar
Cytosar	CYTARABINE
Daktarin	MICONAZOLE
Dalacin C	CLINDAMYCIN
Dalmane	FLURAZEPAM
DANAZOL	Danol
Daneral SA	PHENIRAMINE
Danol	DANAZOL
Dantrium	DANTROLENE
DANTROLENE	Dantrium
Daonil	GLIBENCLAMIDE
DEBRISOQUINE	Declinax
Decadron	DEXAMETHASONE
Declinax	DEBRISOQUINE
Deltacortril	PREDNISOLONE
Deltastab	PREDNISOLONE
De-Nol	BISMUTH CHELATE
De-Noltab	BISMUTH CHELATE
DEOXYCORTONE	Percorten

Proprietary – Generic Drugs

Depixol	FLUPENTHIXOL DECANOATE
Depo-Medrone	METHYLPREDNISOLONE
Dermovate	CLOBETASOL CREAM/OINTMENT
Deseril	METHYSERGIDE
DESIPRAMINE	Pertofran
Destolit	URSODEOXYCHOLIC ACID
DEXAMETHASONE	Decadron, Oradexon
DEXTROMORAMIDE	Palfium
DEXTROPROPOXYPHENE	Doloxene, Cosalgesic*, Distalgesic*, Napsalgesic*
DF 118	DIHYDROCODEINE
Diabinese	CHLORPROPAMIDE
Diamicron	GLICLAZIDE
Diamox	ACETAZOLAMIDE
Diatensec	SPIRONOLACTONE
DIAZEPAM	Alupram, Atensine, Diazemuls (inj), Evacalm, Stesolid (rectal), Valium, Valrelease
DICHLORALPHENAZONE	Welldorm
Diazemuls	DIAZEPAM
DIAZOXIDE	Eudemine
DICLOFENAC	Voltarol
Diconal*	DIPIPANONE/CYCLIZINE
DICYCLOMINE	Merbentyl
Difflam	BENZYDAMINE
DIFLUNISAL	Dolobid
DIGOXIN	Lanoxin
Dihydergot	DIHYDROERGOTAMINE
DIHYDROCODEINE	DF 118, Paramol*
DIHYDROERGOTAMINE	Dihydergot
Dijex*	ALUMINIUM/MAGNESIUM
Dimelor	ACETOHEXAMIDE
DIMETHINDENE	Fenostil, Vibrocil
Dimotane*	BROMPHENIRAMINE/ PSEUDOEPHEDRINE/CODEINE
Dindevan	PHENINDIONE
Dioderm	HYDROCORTISONE
DIPHENHYDRAMINE	Benadryl
DIPHENOXYLATE (with Atropine)	Lomotil*
DIPHENYLPYRALINE	Histryl, Lergoban
DIPIPANONE (with Cyclizine)	Diconal*
Diprosone	BETAMETHASONE

DIPYRIDAMOLE	Persantin
Dirythmin	DISOPYRAMIDE
Disalcid	SALSALATE
Disipal	ORPHENADRINE
DISOPYRAMIDE	Dirythmin, Rythmodan
Distaclor	CEFACLOR
Distalgesic*	DEXTROPROPOXYPHENE/ PARACETAMOL
Distamine	PENICILLAMINE
Distaquaine VK	PENICILLIN V
DISULFIRAM	Antabuse
DITHRANOL	Dithrocream, Psoradrate
Dithrocream	DITHRANOL
Diurexan	XIPAMIDE
Dixarit	CLONIDINE (migraine dose)
DOBUTAMINE	Dobutrex
Dobutrex	DOBUTAMINE
Dolobid	DIFLUNISAL
Doloxene	DEXTROPROPOXYPHENE
Domical	AMITRIPTYLINE
DOMPERIDONE	Motilium
Dopamet	METHYLDOPA
Dormonoct	LOPRAZOLAM
DOTHIEPIN	Prothiaden
Doxatet	DOXYCYCLINE
DOXEPIN	Sinequan
DOXORUBICIN	Adriamycin
DOXYCYCLINE	Doxatet, Doxylar, Vibramycin
Doxylar	DOXYCYCLINE
Droleptan	DROPERIDOL
Dromoran	LEVORPHANOL
DROPERIDOL	Droleptan
Droxalin*	ALUMINIUM/MAGNESIUM
Dryptal	FRUSEMIDE
Dulcolax	BISACODYL
Duogastrone	CARBENOXOLONE
Duphalac	LACTULOSE
Duromorph	MORPHINE
Dytac	TRIAMTERENE

Edecrin	ETHACRYNIC ACID
Efcortelan	HYDROCORTISONE
Efcortesol	HYDROCORTISONE
Efudix	FLUOROURACIL
Elantan	ISOSORBIDE MONONITRATE
Eldepryl	SELEGILINE
Eldisine	VINDESINE
Eltroxin	THYROXINE
Elyzol	METRONIDAZOLE
EMEPRONIUM	Cetiprin
Emeside	ETHOSUXIMIDE
Endoxana	CYCLOPHOSPHAMIDE
Epanutin	PHENYTOIN
Epilim	SODIUM VALPROATE
Equagesic*	ETHOHEPTAZINE/MEPROBAMATE/ ASPIRIN/CALCIUM
Equanil	MEPROBAMATE
Eraldin	PRACTOLOL
ERGOTAMINE	Lingraine, Medihaler ergotamine
Ermysin	ERYTHROMYCIN
Erycen	ERYTHROMYCIN
Erythrocin	ERYTHROMYCIN (STEARATE)
Erythromid	ERYTHROMYCIN
ERYTHROMYCIN	Ermysin, Erycen, Erythrocin, Erythromid, Erythroped, Ilosone, Ilotycin
Erythroped	ERYTHROMYCIN (ETHYL SUCCINATE)
Esbatal	BETHANIDINE
ETHACRYNIC ACID	Edecrin
ETHAMBUTOL	Myambutol
ETHOSUXIMIDE	Emeside, Zarontin
ETOPOSIDE	Vepesid
Eudemine	DIAZOXIDE
Euglucon	GLIBENCLAMIDE
Eugynon*	NORGESTREL/ETHINYLOESTRADIOL
Euhypnos	TEMAZEPAM
Eumovate	CLOBETASONE CREAM/OINTMENT
Evacalm	DIAZEPAM
Exirel	PIRBUTEROL
Fabahistin	MEBHYDROLIN
Feldene	PIROXICAM

Fenbid	IBUPROFEN
FENBUFEN	Lederfen
FENFLURAMINE	Ponderax
FENOPROFEN	Fenopron, Progesic
Fenopron	FENOPROFEN
Fenostil	DIMETHINDENE
FENOTEROL	Berotec
Fentazin	PERPHENAZINE
Feospan	FERROUS SULPHATE
Ferro-Gradumet	FERROUS SULPHATE
FERROUS FUMARATE	Fersamal, Fersaday
FERROUS FUMARATE AND FOLIC ACID	Pregaday
FERROUS SULPHATE	Feospan, Ferrogradumet
Fersaday	FERROUS FUMARATE
Fersamal	FERROUS FUMARATE
Flagyl	METRONIDAZOLE
FLAVOXATE	Urispas
FLECAINIDE	Tambocor
Florinef	FLUDROCORTISONE
Floxapen	FLUCLOXACILLIN
Fluanxol	FLUPENTHIXOL
FLUCLOXACILLIN	Floxapen, Ladropen, Stafoxil
FLUCYTOSINE	Alcobon
FLUDROCORTISONE	Florinef
FLUNITRAZEPAM	Rohypnol
FLUOROURACIL	Efudix
Fluothane	HALOTHANE
FLUPENTHIXOL	Depixol, Fluanxol
FLUPHENAZINE	Modecate, Moditen
FLURAZEPAM	Dalmane
FLURBIPROFEN	Froben
Fortral	PENTAZOCINE
Fortunan	HALOPERIDOL
FRANGULA WITH STERCULIA	Normacol standard (and 'sugar-free')
Frisium	CLOBAZAM
Froben	FLURBIPROFEN
FRUSEMIDE	Alizine, Dryptal, Frumil*, Frusene*, Frusid, Lasipressin, Lasix
Frusene*	FRUSEMIDE/TRIAMTERENE
Frusid	FRUSEMIDE
Fucidin	SODIUM FUSIDATE, FUSIDIC ACID

Fulcin	GRISEOFULVIN
Fungilin	AMPHOTERICIN (topical)
Fungizone	AMPHOTERICIN (oral)
Furadantin	NITROFURANTOIN
FUSIDIC ACID	Fucidin
Fybogel	ISPAGHULA
Fybogel Orange	ISPAGHULA
Fybranta	BRAN
Ganda*	GUANETHIDINE/ADRENALINE
Garamycin	GENTAMICIN
Gardenal	PHENOBARBITONE
Gastrocote*	ALUMINIUM/MAGNESIUM/ALGINIC ACID/SODIUM BICARBONATE
Gastrozepin	PIRENZEPINE
Gatinar	LACTULOSE
Gaviscon*	ALUMINIUM/MAGNESIUM/ALGINATE/ SODIUM BICARBONATE
Gelusil*	ALUMINIUM/MAGNESIUM
GENTAMICIN	Cidomycin, Garamycin, Genticin
Genticin	GENTAMICIN
GLIBENCLAMIDE	Daonil, Euglucon, Libanil, Malix, Semi-Daonil
Glibenese	GLIPIZIDE
GLICLAZIDE	Diamicron
GLIPIZIDE	Glibenese
GLIQUIDONE	Glurenorm
Glucophage	METFORMIN
Glurenorm	GLIQUIDONE
GLYCERYL TRINITRATE	Coro-Nitro Spray, GTN, Nitrocontin, Nitrolingual, Percutol, Suscard, Suscard Buccal, Sustac, Transiderm-Nitro, Tridil
GLYMIDINE	Gondafon
Gondafon	GLYMIDINE
GRISEOFULVIN	Fulcin, Grizovin
Grizovin	GRISEOFULVIN
GTN	GLYCERYL TRINITRATE
GUANETHIDINE	Ganda*, Ismelin
Guanimycin*	DIHYDROSTREPTOMYCIN/SULPHA-GUANIDINE/KAOLIN
Gyno-Daktarin	MICONAZOLE

Halcion	TRIAZOLAM
Haldol	HALOPERIDOL
HALOPERIDOL	Fortunan, Haldol
HALOTHANE	Fluothane
Heminevrin	CHLORMETHIAZOLE
Hismanal	ASTEMIZOLE
Histryl	DIPHENYLPYRALINE
HYDRALAZINE	Apresoline
Hydrea	HYDROXYUREA
HYDROCORTISONE	Colifoam, Corlan, Cortenema, Efcortesol, Efcortelan, Hydrocortistab, Solu-Cortef
HYDROCORTISONE CREAM/OINTMENT	Dioderm
Hydrocortistab	HYDROCORTISONE
HYDROXOCOBALAMIN	Neo-Cytamen
HYDROXYCHLOROQUINE	Plaquenil
HYDROXYUREA	Hydrea
HYOSCINE	Buscopan, 'Kwells'
Hypovase	PRAZOSIN
HYPROMELLOSE	Isopto alkaline, Isopto plain
IBUPROFEN	Apsifen, Brufen, Fenbid, Motrin
Ilosone	ERYTHROMYCIN (ESTOLATE)
Ilotycin	ERYTHROMYCIN
Imbrilon	INDOMETHACIN
Imferon	IRON DEXTRAN
IMIPRAMINE	Tofranil
Imodium	LOPERAMIDE
Imperacin	OXYTETRACYCLINE
Imuran	AZATHIOPRINE
INDAPAMIDE	Natrilix
Inderal	PROPRANOLOL
Indocid	INDOMETHACIN
Indolar	INDOMETHACIN
INDOMETHACIN	Imbrilon, Indocid, Indolar
INDORAMIN	Baratol
Integrin	OXYPERTINE
Ipral	TRIMETHOPRIM
IPRATROPIUM	Atrovent
IRON	see FERROUS salts Imferon (IRON DEXTRAN) Jectofer (IRON SORBITOL/CITRIC ACID COMPLEX) Niferex (IRON POLYSACCHARIDE COMPLEX)

Ismelin	GUANETHIDINE
Ismo	ISOSORBIDE MONONITRATE
Iso-Autohaler	ISOPRENALINE
Isoket	ISOSORBIDE DINITRATE
ISONIAZID	Rimifon
ISOPRENALINE	Iso-Autohaler, Medihaler-Iso, Saventrine
Isopto alkaline	HYPROMELLOSE
Isopto plain	HYPROMELLOSE
Isordil	ISOSORBIDE DINITRATE
ISOSORBIDE DINITRATE	Cedocard, Isoket, Isordil, Soni-Slo, Sotard SA, Sorbichew, Sorbitrate
ISOSORBIDE MONONITRATE	Elantan, Ismo, Monit, Mono-Cedocard
ISPAGHULA	Fybogel
Jectofer	IRON SORBITOL/CITRIC ACID COMPLEX
KANAMYCIN	Kannasyn, Kantrex
Kannasyn	KANAMYCIN
Kantrex	KANAMYCIN
Kaodene*	CODEINE/KAOLIN
KAOLIN MIXTURE	Guanimycin*, Kaodene*
KAOLIN/PECTIN	Kaopectate*
Kaopectate*	KAOLIN/PECTIN
Kefadol	CEPHAMANDOLE
Keflex	CEPHALEXIN
Keflin	CEPHALOTHIN
Kefzol	CEPHAZOLIN
Kemadrin	PROCYCLIDINE
Kemicetine	CHLORAMPHENICOL
Kenalog	TRIAMCINOLONE
KETAZOLAM	Anxon
KETOCONAZOLE	Nizoral
KETOPROFEN	Alrheumat, Orudis, Oruvail
KETOTIFEN	Zaditen
Kiditard	QUINIDINE
Kinidin	QUINIDINE
LABETALOL	Trandate
LACTULOSE	Duphalac, Gatinar
Ladropen	FLUCLOXACILLIN
Lanoxin	DIGOXIN
Lanvis	THIOGUANINE

Proprietary – Generic Drugs

Larodopa	LEVODOPA
Laratrim	CO-TRIMOXAZOLE
Largactil	CHLORPROMAZINE
Lasipressin*	FRUSEMIDE/PENBUTOLOL
Lasix	FRUSEMIDE
Lasma	THEOPHYLLINE
LATAMOXEF	Moxalactam
Ledercort	TRIAMCINOLONE
Lederfen	FENBUFEN
Lederspan	TRIAMCINOLONE (inj)
Lentizol	AMITRIPTYLINE
Lergoban	DIPHENYLPYRALINE
Leukeran	CHLORAMBUCIL
Levius	ASPIRIN
LEVODOPA	Brocadopa, Larodopa, Madopar*, Sinemet*, Sinemet-Plus*
LEVONORGESTREL COMBINATIONS	Cyclo-progynova, Eugynon, Logynon, Microgynon, Neogest, Norgeston, Schering PC4
LEVORPHANOL	Dromoran
Lexotan	BROMAZEPAM
Libanil	GLIBENCLAMIDE
Librium	CHLORDIAZEPOXIDE
LIDOFLAZINE	Clinium
LIGNOCAINE	Lignostab, Xylocaine, Xylocard
Lignostab	LIGNOCAINE
Lincocin	LINCOMYCIN
Lingraine	ERGOTAMINE
LINCOMYCIN	Lincocin
Lioresal	BACLOFEN
LIQUID PARAFFIN/ MAGNESIUM HYDROXIDE	Milpar*
Liskonium	LITHIUM CARBONATE
Litarex	LITHIUM CITRATE
LITHIUM CARBONATE	Camcolit, Liskonum, Phasal, Priadel
LITHIUM CITRATE	Litarex
Logynon*	ETHINYLOESTRADIOL/LEVO-NORGESTREL
Lomotil*	DIPHENOXYLATE/ATROPINE
Loniten	MINOXIDIL
LOPERAMIDE	Imodium
LOPRAZOLAM	Dormonoct
Lopressor	METOPROLOL

Loramet	LORMETAZEPAM
LORAZEPAM	Almazine, Ativan
LORMETAZEPAM	Loramet, Noctamid
Ludiomil	MAPROTILINE
Luminal	PHENOBARBITONE
Macrodantin	NITROFURANTOIN
Madopar*	LEVODOPA/BENSERAZIDE
MAGNESIUM/ALUMINIUM	Aludrox*, Dijex*, Gelusil*, Polycrol*, Polycrol Forte*, Prodexin*, Topal*
MAGNESIUM TRISILICATE	APP*, Droxalin*, Gaviscon*, Gastrocote*, Gelusil*, Nulacin*, Pyrogastrone*
Malix	GLIBENCLAMIDE
MAPROTILINE	Ludiomil
Maxolon	METOCLOPRAMIDE
MAZINDOL	Teronac
MEBEVERINE	Colofac
MEBHYDROLIN	Fabahistin
MEDAZEPAM	Nobrium
Medihaler-Ergotamine	ERGOTAMINE
Medihaler-Iso	ISOPRENALINE
Medrone	METHYLPREDNISOLONE
MEFENAMIC ACID	Ponstan
Mefoxin	CEFOXITIN
MEFRUSIDE	Baycaron
Melitase	CHLORPROPAMIDE
Melleril	THIORIDAZINE
MELPHALAN	Alkeran
MEPROBAMATE	Equagesic*, Equanil, Tenavoid*
MEPTAZINOL	Meptid
Meptid	MEPTAZINOL
MEPYRAMINE	Anthisan
Merbentyl	DICYCLOMINE
MERCAPTOPURINE	Puri-Nethol
Merital	NOMIFENSINE
Metenix	METOLAZONE
METFORMIN	Glucophage
METHADONE	Physeptone
METHOTRIMEPRAZINE	Nozinan, Veractil
METHYLDOPA	Aldomet, Dopamet
METHYLPHENIDATE	Ritalin

METHYLPREDNISOLONE	Depo-Medrone, Medrone, Neo-Medrone, Solu-Medrone
METHYSERGIDE	Deseril
METOCLOPRAMIDE	Maxolon, Metox, Parmid, Primperan
METOLAZONE	Metenix
METOPROLOL	Betaloc, Lopressor
Metox	METOCLOPRAMIDE
Metrolyl	METRONIDAZOLE
METRONIDAZOLE	Elyzol, Flagyl, Metrolyl, Nidazol, Zadstat
MEXILETINE	Mexitel
Mexitel	MEXILETINE
MEZLOCILLIN	Baypen
MIANSERIN	Bolvidon, Norval
MICONAZOLE	Daktarin, Dormonistat, Gyno-Daktarin, Monistat
Microgynon*	NORGESTREL/ETHINYLOESTRADIOL
Micronor	NORETHISTERONE
Midamor	AMILORIDE
'Mil-par'*	MAGNESIUM HYDROXIDE/LIQUID PARAFFIN
Minocin	MINOCYCLINE
MINOCYCLINE	Minocin
MINOXIDIL	Loniten
Modecate	FLUPHENAZINE
Moditen	FLUPHENAZINE
Mogadon	NITRAZEPAM
Molipaxin	TRAZODONE
Monaspor	CEFSULODIN
Monistat	MICONAZOLE
Monit	ISOSORBIDE MONONITRATE
Mono-Cedocard	ISOSORBIDE MONONITRATE
Monotrim	TRIMETHOPRIM
MORPHINE	Duromorph, MST-Continus, Nepenthe
Motilium	IMODIUM
Moxalactam	LATAMOXEF
MST-Continus	MORPHINE
Myambutol	ETHAMBUTOL
Mycardol	PENTAERYTHRITOL TETRANITRATE
Mycifradin	NEOMYCIN
Myleran	BUSULPHAN
Mysoline	PRIMIDONE

Proprietary — Generic Drugs

NABILONE	Cesamet
NADOLOL	Corgard
NALIDIXIC ACID	Negram
NALOXONE	Narcan
Naprosyn	NAPROXEN
NAPROXEN	Naprosyn, Synflex
Napsalgesic*	DEXTROPROPOXYPHENE/PARA-CETAMOL
Narcan	NALOXONE
Nardil	PHENELZINE
Narphen	PHENAZOCINE
Natrilix	INDAPAMIDE
Natulan	PROCARBAZINE
Nebcin	TOBRAMYCIN
NEFOPAM	Acupan
Negram	NALIDIXIC ACID
Neo-Cytamen	HYDROXOCOBALAMIN
Neogest	NORGESTREL
Neo-Medrone*	METHYLPREDNISOLONE/NEOMYCIN/ALUMINIUM/SULPHUR
Neo-Mercazole	CARBIMAZOLE
NEOMYCIN	Mycifradin, Nivemycin
Neo-Na Clex	BENDROFLUAZIDE
Neoplatin	CISPLATIN
NEOSTIGMINE	Prostigmin
Nepenthe	OPIUM ALKALOIDS
Netillin	NETILMICIN
NETILMICIN	Netillin
Neutradonna*	ALUMINIUM/BELLADONNA
Nidazol	METRONIDAZOLE
NIFEDIPINE	Adalat
Niferex	IRON SORBITOL COMPLEX
Nitrados	NITRAZEPAM
NITRAZEPAM	Mogadon, Nitrados, Somnite
Nitrocontin	GLYCERYL TRINITRATE
Nitrolingual	GLYCERYL TRINITRATE
NITROFURANTOIN	Berkfurin, Furadantin, Macrodantin
Nivaquine	CHLOROQUINE
Nivemycin	NEOMYCIN
Nizoral	KETOCONAZOLE
Nobrium	MEDAZEPAM
Noctamid	LORMETAZEPAM

Noctec	CHLORAL HYDRATE
Nolvadex	TAMOXIFEN
NOMIFENSINE	Merital
NORETHISTERONE	Micronor, Noriday, Noristerat, Primolut N, Utovlan
Norflex	ORPHENADRINE
Norgeston	LEVONORGESTREL
Noriday	NORETHISTERONE
Noristerat	NORETHISTERONE OENANTHATE
Normacol standard* (and sugar free)	STERCULIA/FRANGULA
Normison	TEMAZEPAM
NORTRIPTYLINE	Allegron, Aventyl
Norval	MIANSERIN
Nozinan	METHOTRIMEPRAZINE
Nu-Seal Aspirin (enteric coated)	ASPIRIN
Nuelin	THEOPHYLLINE
Nulacin*	MILK POWDER/MAGNESIUM/CALCIUM CARBONATE
Nystan	NYSTATIN
NYSTATIN	Nystan, Nystavescent
Nystavescent	NYSTATIN
Ocusert	PILOCARPINE
OESTROGENS	Premarin, Prempak-C
Oncovin	VINCRISTINE
Optimax	TRYPTOPHAN
Optimine	AZATADINE
Oradexon	DEXAMETHASONE
Orap	PIMOZIDE
Orbenin	CLOXACILLIN
ORCIPRENALINE	Alupent
Orimeten	AMINOGLUTETHIMIDE
ORPHENADRINE	Disipal, Norflex
Orudis	KETOPROFEN
Oruvail	KETOPROFEN
Ospolot	SULTHIAME
Otrivine-Antistin*	XYLOMETAZOLINE/ANTAZOLINE
OXATOMIDE	Tinset
OXAZEPAM	Serenid D
OXPRENOLOL	Apsolox, Slow-Trasicor, Trasicor
OXYPERTINE	Integrin

Proprietary — Generic Drugs

265

OXYPHENBUTAZONE	Tanderil
OXYTETRACYCLINE	Berkmycen, Imperacin, Terramycin
Pacitron	TRYPTOPHAN
Palfium	DEXTROMORAMIDE
Paludrine	PROGUANIL
Panadol	PARACETAMOL
Panasorb	PARACETAMOL
PARACETAMOL	Calpol, Panadol, Panasorb
Parlodel	BROMOCRIPTINE
Parmid	METOCLOPRAMIDE
Parnate	TRANYLCYPROMINE
Penbritin	AMPICILLIN
PENBUTALOL/FRUSEMIDE	Lasipressin*
Pendramine	PENICILLAMINE
PENICILLAMINE	Distamine, Pendramine
PENICILLIN V	Apsin VK, Crystapen V, Stabilin V-K, V-Cil-K
PENTAERYTHRITOL TETRANITRATE	Cardiacap, Mycardol, Peritrate
PENTAZOCINE	Fortral
Percorten	DEOXYCORTONE
Percutol	GLYCERYL TRINITRATE
Periactin	CYPROHEPTADINE
Peritrate	PENTAERYTHRITOL TETRANITRATE
PERPHENAZINE	Fentazin
Persantin	DIPYRIDAMOLE
Pertofran	DESIPRAMINE
Phasal	LITHIUM CARBONATE
PHENAZOCINE	Narphen
PHENELZINE	Nardil
Phenergan	PROMETHAZINE
PHENINDIONE	Dindevan
PHENIRAMINE	Daneral SA
PHENOBARBITONE	Gardenal, Luminal
PHENOLPHTHALEIN	Agarol*, Alophen*, Veracolate*
PHENOXYMETHYL PENICILLIN	see PENICILLIN V
PHENYTOIN	Epanutin
Phyllocontin	AMINOPHYLLINE
Physeptone	METHADONE
PILOCARPINE	Ocusert, Sno Pilo

PIMOZIDE	Orap
PINDOLOL	Visken
PIPERACILLIN	Pipril
Pipril	PIPERACILLIN
PIRBUTEROL	Exirel
PIRENZEPINE	Gastrozepin
Piriton	CHLORPHENIRAMINE
PIROXICAM	Feldene
PIZOTIFEN	Sanomigran
Plaquenil	HYDROXYCHLOROQUINE
Platinex	CISPLATIN
Polycrol*	ALUMINIUM/MAGNESIUM/ DIMETHICONE
POLYMIXIN	Aerosporin
Ponderax	FENFLURAMINE
Ponstan	MEFENAMIC ACID
PRACTOLOL	Eraldin
Pramidex	TOLBUTAMIDE
PRAZEPAM	Centrax
PRAZOSIN	Hypovase
Prednesol	PREDNISOLONE
PREDNISOLONE	Codelsol, Deltacortril (enteric coated), Deltastab, Prednesol, Predsol, Sintisone
PREDNISOLONE EYE DROPS	Predsol
Predsol	PREDNISOLONE EYE DROPS
Pregaday*	FERROUS FUMARATE/FOLIC ACID
Premarin	CONJUGATED OESTROGENS
Prempak-C*	CONJUGATED OESTROGENS/ NORGESTREL
PRENYLAMINE	Synadrin
Priadel	LITHIUM CARBONATE
PRIMIDONE	Mysoline
Primolut N	NORETHISTERONE
Primoteston Depot	TESTOSTERONE OENANTHATE
Primperan	METOCLOPRAMIDE
Pro-Actidil	TRIPROLIDINE
Pro-Banthine	PROPANTHELINE
PROBENECID	Benemid
PROCAINAMIDE	Pronestyl
PROCARBAZINE	Natulan
PROCHLORPERAZINE	Stemetil, Vertigon

Proprietary – Generic Drugs

PROCYCLIDINE	Kemadrin
Prodexin*	ALUMINIUM/MAGNESIUM
Progesic	FENOPROFEN
PROGUANIL	Paludrine
PROMETHAZINE	Avomine, Phenergan
Pronestyl	PROCAINAMIDE
PROPANTHELINE	Pro-Banthine
PROPRANOLOL	Apsolol, Berkolol, Inderal
Prostigmin	NEOSTIGMINE
Prothiaden	DOTHIEPIN
PROTRIPTYLINE	Concordin
Pro-Vent	THEOPHYLLINE
PSEUDOEPHEDRINE	Sudafed SA
Psoradrate	DITHRANOL
Pulmadil	RIMITEROL
Pulmicort	BUDESONIDE
Puri-Nethol	MERCAPTOPURINE
Pyopen	CARBENICILLIN
PYRAZINAMIDE	Zinamide
Pyrogastrone*	CARBENOXOLONE/ALUMINIUM/ MAGNESIUM/SODIUM ALGINATE/ POTASSIUM BICARBONATE
Questran	CHOLESTYRAMINE
QUINIDINE	Kiditard, Kinidin
RANITIDINE	Zantac
Rastinon	TOLBUTAMIDE
Redoxon	ASCORBIC ACID
REPROTEROL	Bronchodil
RESERPINE	Abicol, Seominal*
Restandol	TESTOSTERONE UNDECANOATE
Rheumox	AZAPROPAZONE
Rifadin	RIFAMPICIN
RIFAMPICIN	Rifadin, Rimactane
Rimactane	RIFAMPICIN
Rimifon	ISONIAZID
RIMITEROL	Pulmadil
Ritalin	METHYLPHENIDATE
Rivotril	CLONAZEPAM
Ro-A-Vit	VITAMIN A
Rohypnol	FLUNITRAZEPAM

Roscorbic	ASCORBIC ACID
Rythmodan	DISOPYRAMIDE
Salazopyrin	SULPHASALAZINE
Salbulin	SALBUTAMOL
SALBUTAMOL	Asmaven, Salbulin, Ventolin
SALSALATE	Disalcid
Saluric	CHLOROTHIAZIDE
Sandimmun	CYCLOSPORIN
Sanomigran	PIZOTIFEN
Saventrine	ISOPRENALINE
Schering PC 4*	LEVONORGESTREL/ETHINYL-OESTRADIOL
Sectral	ACEBUTOLOL
Securopen	AZLOCILLIN
SELEGILINE	Eldepryl
Semi-Daonil	GLIBENCLAMIDE
Seominal*	RESERPINE/PHENOBARITONE/THEOBROMINE
Septrin	CO-TRIMOXAZOLE
Serc	BETAHISTINE
Serenid D	OXAZEPAM
Serophene	CLOMIPHENE
Siloxyl*	ALUMINIUM/MAGNESIUM/DIMETHICONE
Sinequan	DOXEPIN
Sinemet*, Sinemet-Plus*	LEVODOPA/CARBIDOPA
Sintisone	PREDNISOLONE
Slo-Phyllin	THEOPHYLLINE
Slow-Trasicor	OXPRENOLOL
Sno Phenicol	CHLORAMPHENICOL EYE DROPS
Sno Pilo	PILOCARPINE EYE DROPS
SODIUM FUSIDATE	Fucidin
SODIUM VALPROATE	Epilim
Solprin	ASPIRIN
Solu-Cortef	HYDROCORTISONE
Solu-Medrone	METHYLPREDNISOLONE
Somnite	NITRAZEPAM
Soni-Slo	ISOSORBIDE DINITRATE
Sorbichew	ISOSORBIDE DINITRATE
Sorbitrate	ISOSORBIDE DINITRATE
Sotacor	SOTALOL

SOTALOL	Beta-Cardone, Sotacor
Sotard SA	ISOSORBIDE DINITRATE
Spiroctan	SPIRONOLACTONE
Spirolone	SPIRONOLACTONE
SPIRONOLACTONE	Aldactone, Diatensec, Spiroctan, Spirolone
Stabilin VK	PENICILLIN V
Stadol	BUTORPHANOL
Stafoxyl	FLUCLOXACILLIN
STANOZOLOL	Stromba
Stelazine	TRIFLUOPERAZINE
Stemetil	PROCHLORPERAZINE
Stesolid	DIAZEPAM
Stromba	STANOZOLOL
Stugeron	CINNARIZINE
SUCRALFATE	Antepsin
Sudafed SA	PSEUDOEPHEDRINE
SULINDAC	Clinoril
SULPHADIMIDINE	Sulphamethazethine
SULPHAMETHAZONE	Urolucosil
Sulphamezathine	SULPHADIMIDINE
SULPHASALAZINE	Salazopyrin
SULPHINPYRAZONE	Anturan
SULTHIAME	Ospolot
Suscard, Suscard Buccal	GLYCERYL TRINITRATE
Sustac	GLYCERYL TRINITRATE
Sustanon	TESTOSTERONE
Symmetrel	AMANTADINE
Tagamet	CIMETIDINE
Tambocor	FLECAINIDE
Tamofen	TAMOXIFEN
TAMOXIFEN	Nolvadex, Tamofen
Tanderil	OXYPHENBUTAZONE
Tavegil	CLEMASTINE
Tegretol	CARBAMAZEPINE
TEMAZEPAM	Euhypnos, Normison
Temgesic	BUPRENORPHINE
Tenavoid*	BENDROFLUAZIDE/MEPROBAMATE
TERBUTALINE	Bricanyl
TERFENADINE	Triludan
Teronac	MAZINDOL

Terramycin	OXYTETRACYCLINE
Testoral	TESTOSTERONE
TESTOSTERONE	Restandol, Sustanon, Testoral, Virormone
TETRACYCLINE	Achromycin, Sustamycin, Tetrabid, Tetrachel, Tetrex
TETRACYCLINE OINTMENT	Achromycin
Theo-Dur	THEOPHYLLINE
Theograd	THEOPHYLLINE
THEOPHYLLINE	Lasma, Nuelin, Pro-Vent, Slo-Phyllin, Theo-Dur, Theograd, Uniphyllin
THIOGUANINE	Lanvis
THIORIDAZINE	Melleril
THYROXINE	Eltroxin
TIAPROFENIC ACID	Surgam
Ticar	TICARCILLIN
TICARCILLIN	Ticar
TIMOLOL	Betim, Blocadren, Timoptol
Timoptol	TIMOLOL
TIMOLOL EYE DROPS	Timoptol
Tinset	OXATOMIDE
Tobralex	TOBRAMYCIN EYE DROPS
TOBRAMYCIN	Nebcin, Tobralex
TOCAINIDE	Tonocard
Tofranil	IMIPRAMINE
Tolanase	TOLAZAMIDE
TOLAZAMIDE	Tolanase
Tolectin	TOLMETIN
TOLBUTAMIDE	Pramidex, Rastinon
TOLMETIN	Tolectin
Tonocard	TOCAINIDE
Topal*	ALUMINIUM/MAGNESIUM
Transiderm-Nitro	GLYCERYL TRINITRATE
Tranxene	CLORAZEPATE
TRANYLCYPROMINE	Parnate
Trasicor	OXPRENOLOL
TRAZODONE	Molipaxin
TRIAMCINOLONE	Adcortyl, Kenalog, Ledercort, Lederspan
TRIAMTERENE	Dytac, Frusent
TRIAZOLAM	Halcion
Tridil	GLYCERYL TRINITRATE
TRIFLUOPERAZINE	Stelazine
Triludan	TERFENADINE

TRIMEPRAZINE	Vallergan
TRIMETHOPRIM	Ipral, Monotrim, Syraprim, Trimopan
Trimopan	TRIMETHOPRIM
TRI-POTASSIUM DI-CITRATO BISMUTHATE	see BISMUTH CHELATE
TRIPROLIDINE	Actidil, Pro-Actidil
TRYPTOPHAN	Pacitron, Optimax
Tryptizol	AMITRIPTYLINE
Uniphyllin	THEOPHYLLINE
Urispas	FLAVOXATE
Urolucosil	SULPHAMETHIZOLE
URSODEOXYCHOLIC ACID	Destolet
Utovlan	NORETHISTERONE
Valium	DIAZEPAM
Vallergan	TRIMEPRAZINE
Valoid	Cyclizine
Valrelease	DIAZEPAM
Vancocin	VANCOMYCIN
VANCOMYCIN	Vancocin
V-Cil-K	PENICILLIN V
Velosef	CEPHRADINE
Ventolin	SALBUTAMOL
Vepesid	ETOPOSIDE
Veracolate*	PHENOLPHTHALEIN/CASCARA/BILE SALTS
Veractil	METHOTRIMEPRAZINE
VERAPAMIL	Berkatens, Cordilox, Securon
Vertigon	PROCHLORPERAZINE
Vibramycin	DOXYCYCLINE
Vibrocil*	PHENYLEPHRINE/DIMETHINDENE/NEOMYCIN
VIDARABINE	Vira-A
Vidopen	AMPICILLIN
VILOXAZINE	Vivalan
VINCRISTINE	Oncovin
VINDESINE	Eldisine
Vira-A	VIDARABINE
Virormone	TESTOSTERONE
Visken	PINDOLOL
Vivalen	VILOXAZINE

VITAMIN A	Ro-A-Vit
Voltarol	DICLOFENAC
WARFARIN	Marevan
Welldorm	DICHLORALPHENAZONE
Xanax	ALPRAZOLAM
XIPAMIDE	Diurexan
Xylocard	LIGNOCAINE
Xylocaine	LIGNOCAINE
Zaditen	KETOTIFEN
Zadstat	METRONIDAZOLE
Zantac	RANITIDINE
Zarontin	ETHOSUXIMIDE
Zinacef	CEFUROXIME
Zinamide	PYRAZINAMIDE
ZINC SULPHATE	Z Span
Zovirax	ACYCLOVIR
Z Span	ZINC SULPHATE
Zyloric	ALLOPURINOL

Index

index

Index

Index

index

Index

index

index

index

index

291

index

Index

PRACTICAL PRESCRIBING

This book is divided into 7 sections. Please indicate your rating of each by circling the appropriate number. Some comment regarding alterations and additions would be appreciated.

Section 1 **Glossary**   POOR   1   2   3   4   EXCELLENT

Alterations:

Additions:

Section 2 **Drugs of choice**   POOR   1   2   3   4   EXCELLENT

Alterations:

Additions:

Section 3 **Drug treatment policies**   POOR   1   2   3   4   EXCELLENT

Alterations:

Additions:

Section 4 **Pharmacological broadsheets**   POOR   1   2   3   4   EXCELLENT

Alterations:

Additions:

Section 5 **Side-effects**   POOR   1   2   3   4   EXCELLENT

Alterations:

Additions:

Section 6 **Drug interactions**   POOR   1   2   3   4   EXCELLENT

Alterations:

Additions:

Section 7 **Cautions**   POOR   1   2   3   4   EXCELLENT

Alterations:

Additions:

More detailed criticism will be welcome.
Please send to: Dr Martin J Brodie
            Clinical Pharmacology Unit
            University Department of Medicine
            Western Infirmary
            Glasgow G11 6NT